behind clinic doors

Emily A. Haynie, PA-C

© 2024 Emily A. Haynie

All rights reserved. No part of this book may be reproduced or transmitted by any means, without the prior written permission of the author.

All patient and healthcare professional names are fictitious, and other recognizable features have been changed. The people portrayed are composites; they may represent several individuals whose characteristics and experiences were adapted and combined to form a character. All events portrayed are factual, although details and timelines may be similarly altered to protect confidentiality and privacy. This book does not constitute medical, legal, or other actionable advice.

Editing by Holly Baker
Cover and book design by Meagan Jeanneret
Photographs from the author's personal collection

The author is grateful for permission to use the following previously copyrighted material: Paul Spiegelman and Britt Berrett, *Patients Come Second: Leading Change by Changing the Way You Lead* (New York: An Inc. Original, 2013).

Library of Congress Control Number: 2024908939
ISBN 979-8332585784

Distributed by Kindle Direct Publishing

Printed in the United States of America

For Matthew

"If we cannot laugh and enjoy the good times, it is hard to handle the inevitable difficult times."

Dane Peterson, *Patients Come Second*

CONTENTS

Prologue   x

PART I | THE STUDENT

Didactic Year: Gross Anatomy	16
Child's Play	24
Didactic Year: Physical Examination	28
Didactic Year: Cultural (In)Competency	32
Wait … I'm Asian?	36
Clinical Year: OB/GYN	42
Clinical Year: Pimpin' Ain't Easy	50
Clinical Year: Emergency Medicine	54
Clinical Year: Surgery	76

PART II | THE EARLY YEARS

Green in a White Coat	88
Learning from the Best	98
The Birds and the Bees	108
How to Be a Professional	116
Family Practice	124
Possible Side Effect: Murder	164
Heartbreak	170
Diego Goes to the Doctor	176
Self-harm via Marine Life	184
For the Living	186

PART III | THE WONDER YEARS

The Spark	194
Crossing the Line	202
What Do You Do for Work?	208

The Hayn Bug	212
Borderline	214
A Mother's Grief	218
HLF	222
Pedobug	228
It's Been a Long Day, to Say the Least	232
Two Honey Buns or Two Almonds?	234
A Father's Misfortune	252
Tug of War	260
Fighting Against the Clock	264
Chart Tetris	270
EMR	276
The Culture of Medicine	284

PART IV | COVID-19

Volcano	290
Earthquake	296
Every Man for Himself	300
False Alarm	306
Brainwashed	308
An Unexpected Discovery	314
Till Death Do Us Part	316
Say "Ahh"	322
Rice Chaser	324
It's Not All in Your Head	332
It's in the Air	338
Staple Him Up	342
Resilience	346

Epilogue	356
Appendix: Photos	363
Acknowledgments	372

PROLOGUE

It's really happening. I took a deep breath as heavy doors opened to a dimly lit auditorium and a hush fell temporarily over the murmuring swell of laughter and chatter on the other side. Almost immediately, it was replaced by clicks and glinting lights from smartphone cameras. As a gust of cool air drifted toward us, I distractedly smoothed out the soft folds of my favorite red dress with the heart-shaped neckline. The last thing I needed was to flash everyone when I made my grand entrance.

We soaked up every moment of our celebrity status as we made our way down the aisle, dressed to the nines in comparison to our usual uniforms of athleisure, casual chic, and T-shirts damp with sweat from the merciless Houston humidity. A year ago, we had converged on Baylor College of Medicine as forty perfect strangers from almost every state. Today's White Coat Ceremony cemented our transition from the academic to the clinical phase of physician assistant (PA) school, when we would see real patients. We had spent every weekday together in the same handful of windowless classrooms. Unlike the hundreds of anonymous students we had shared huge lecture halls with in college, we knew one another intimately. The never-ending drumline of PowerPoints parading before our eyes eight hours a day, the determination to cram our heads full of medical facts with every moment of free time we had, the weeklong blocks of exams every eight weeks a brutal exercise in cognitive and physical stamina ... it was all behind us now. A shared struggle for survival had bonded us as a group. Two of our classmates had dropped out, and several more agonized over whether to stay or to leave due to the program's academic difficulty or to personal challenges. I had questioned on many occasions whether I would be among the final thirty-eight still standing. Not one of us took this moment for granted.

Our families and significant others craned their necks and took photos to memorialize these promising young people. They celebrated as much as we did that Didactic Year was coming to a close; some had moved to Houston with us, some had supported us from a distance, and all had bent over backwards throughout this rollercoaster ride so that we could pursue our calling. They built us up when we felt like it was too hard to keep going; listened to us when we whined, vented, or put ourselves down; and managed to keep the other parts of our lives intact.

My classmates and I proudly donned our short white coats—which signified that we were still students—and listened intently as our professors gave impassioned speeches about the continuous, lifelong pursuit of learning, and the tenacity and bravery that clinical year would demand of us. For our final act, we stood, faced our families, and uttered the Hippocratic oath like a congregation indistinctly murmuring the Lord's Prayer: "I swear to fulfill, to the best of my ability and judgment, this covenant. I will respect the privacy of my patients, for their problems are not disclosed to me that the world may know. Most especially must I tread with care in matters of life and death. ... May I always act so as to preserve the finest traditions of my calling, and may I long experience the joy of healing those who seek my help."

As a few of my classmates really worked the angles in their new attire, the rows of paparazzi blinded us. I couldn't have known that in the near future, my crisp, starched coat would be dripping with a patient's vomit as I put my first ever IV line in. My face would sting with perspiration, and it would take every fiber of my being to ignore the stench and repulsion so I could complete the final task of my twelve-hour overnight shift. I wonder whether any of us fully comprehended the oath we took that day; I know I didn't. I hadn't seen a single real patient yet. I had neither heard their problems nor been tested with matters of life and death. I had not shouldered the simultaneous responsibilities of clinician, advocate, teacher, detective, and confidant. I did not know how bureaucratic challenges and a global pandemic could make me question the healthcare system's priorities or my own compassion and optimism for helping others. In several years' time, some of my classmates would still find their purpose and passion as PAs, while others would move on to different careers.

But the day of the White Coat Ceremony, the future was bright. This was just the beginning of the most anticipated chapter of our lives. I was giddy with pride at completing another difficult step toward becoming Emily, the PA, when I would no longer be just a student, but a colleague of the very people who spoke from the podium before me. I would help ill people become well and healthy people stay well, providing care that so many patients needed. This was what I was meant to do.

PART I

THE STUDENT

DIDACTIC YEAR: GROSS ANATOMY

Everyone's heard of *Grey's Anatomy*, but how many people have heard of Gross Anatomy? I had no idea that Gross Anatomy lab (aka cadaver lab) was part of the required curriculum for PA school and that we would be spending the semester with corpses, studying all the structures visible to the naked eye—"gross" structures. The objective of the course was to ultimately identify every organ, muscle, bone, nerve, ligament, and blood vessel in the human body by sight. But dead people seemed excessive and extreme; couldn't we just learn anatomy from one of those plastic skeletons? I wanted to be a PA so I could take care of living patients, not become a medical examiner.

The first time my classmates and I rode the elevator down to the cadaver lab in the Baylor basement, we were uncharacteristically silent. I guess I wasn't the only one who found the whole prospect unnerving. Rather than feel comforted, though, I thought the anticipation and apprehension was going to make me sick. *Did I have to actually touch the dead body?*

When the elevator stopped, we all involuntarily tensed as if the doors would open to rows of corpses lined up, or zombies emerging from the darkness. I loved horror movies, but at that moment, I felt uncannily like a character walking into one of them. We congregated in a doorway where our anatomy professor introduced the cold, drab dungeon that was to be our classroom. Just beyond him, we could see several metal tables. Each had a thick, blue, plastic body bag on its surface concealing what we knew was a dead body inside. When they were alive, our professor told us, these people had generously chosen to donate their remains after death to further the education of future PAs and physicians. I stared with horror and fascination (but mostly horror) as I stood at this threshold between the living and the dead. These people had entrusted strangers to poke, prod, and mutilate every nook and cranny of their bodies like pumpkins to be carved, all in the name of science. (The official version was that cadaver dissection was the most precise way to learn the complicated structures of the human body and practice surgical skills. I was skeptical.)

This was just about all I remember before the overpowering smell of formaldehyde hit me. Even though we are all regularly exposed to small amounts of formaldehyde in the air from common things like wood products, fabrics, paint, and cigarette smoke, most people will never know that noxious, distinct odor. The only way I can describe the stench is ammonia mixed with wet, rotting carcasses. The concentration of formaldehyde in Gross Anatomy lab was on another level; an invisible wave simultaneously burned my nostrils, soured my mouth, and stung my eyes. Along with my classmates, I silently helped myself to gloves and a disposable plastic apron to wear over my scrubs. I couldn't imagine how I was going to endure the smell to concentrate and learn anything. It felt like my own innards would brown and wilt like a cadaver's if I simply breathed in too deeply.

That first lab session felt interminable. After a few brave souls unzipped the body bags and exposed our assigned cadavers, groups of students huddled awkwardly around the tables. We tried not to gag as we matched the rancid, stringy, brown body parts in front of us to the colorful images in the anatomy textbooks propped open on stands. The most realistic illustrations do not compare with an actual human body. There were no red tendons or blue blood vessels, only body parts that were all the same shade of brown and had the consistency of very dry pulled pork. The toxic odors of embalming chemicals and decay were overwhelming. The professor kept a watchful eye for students who became nauseated or dizzy, helping them into the hallway or a nearby empty classroom for some fresh air. While I managed not to get physically sick, I fought an equally strong urge to turn around and bolt. The only thing that kept me there was knowing that I could kiss my dreams of becoming a PA goodbye if I didn't make it through this class. When the lab session mercifully ended and I returned to my apartment, I peeled off my scrubs like they were diseased and took the longest shower of my life. There was no way I could do this every week.

I owed part of my survival that semester to one of the students in my lab group, Alex. A man of many talents, the greatest of which was his unapologetic sense of humor, Alex always found ways to remind my classmates and me not to take ourselves too seriously.

"Blanche," he said loudly out of nowhere one day. Our group was stooped over our cadaver, our faces nearly an inch away from the pulled pork as we debated whether a brown string was a nerve or a vein.

"What?" I asked, looking up.

"She looks like a Blanche, so that'll be her name from now on," Alex declared, referring to the pale, bloodless gray of our cadaver's skin. The nameless woman had become a familiar presence that my group gathered around every week as if performing some grisly religious ritual. We would not learn our donors' names until the final day of school in a ceremony that honored their contributions to medicine. Despite initial snickers and eye rolls, Alex's moniker stuck.

As the weeks passed, I was surprised to find that I acclimated a little more quickly each time to the pervasive formaldehyde fog. After we studied an assigned body region in the textbook, we explored the same area on our cadavers or on individually preserved torsos, brains, feet, and other body parts that were shared among all the groups. We visualized normal internal structures as well as unexpected findings due to natural human variation, past surgery, and disease. We learned to be patient, gentle, and steady with our cadavers. Obviously, we could not cause pain or paralysis by cutting a nerve or an artery, but one quick movement could obscure a structure's relationship to the others. Even I eventually conceded that a plastic skeleton model could never offer the same intimate look at the anatomical landmarks referenced in physical examination techniques and therapeutic procedures. There were no computers, cell phones, or other technologies—just the living learning from the dead.

I'm not saying it ever felt natural to be in that basement; no, I never got used to that freezing cold, windowless chamber of death and decay. Unlike other students, I never once went alone to study when the lab was open after hours. (I probably would have made a better grade if I had.) Perhaps horror movies had caused irreparable damage to my imagination, but I occasionally still had the sensation that if I turned my back on one of the bodies, it would somehow come back alive. The amount of formaldehyde I inhaled each week also already seemed more than adequate. Thus, I made the most that I could out of group lab time.

Alex knew I was an easy target. We had started the semester by examining the structures in our cadaver's feet, uncovering a little more of the body in subsequent sessions as we gradually worked our way up towards her head. All the cadavers laid on their backs. Their faces, covered with towels, remained hidden until the final weeks. Alex always managed to pick the perfect moment to grab my arm and exclaim, "Emily, did you see that? I think Blanche's face covering just moved a little," then cackle wickedly as I jumped a foot. Once, as I bent over to inspect a muscle in Blanche's thigh, Alex saw an opportunity he couldn't pass up and moved her lifeless hand so that it brushed against my scrubs. No learning occurred for the next five minutes as I regained my composure.

Occasionally, classmates discovered an anomaly or a retained object in their cadavers.

"What is *that*?" a classmate cried one afternoon from across the room. We were studying the pelvic cavity, and he pointed at something in his male cadaver with his forceps, inadvertently sending a bit of decayed human flesh onto the greasy anatomy book beside him. The professor wandered over, took a quick look, and laughed mischievously.

"Here we have a well-preserved vacuum constriction device," he said didactically. "Does anyone know the generic term?"

"Penis pump," one of the guys said casually.

"Yes, a penis pump," the professor repeated in his loud, booming voice while several classmates giggled like teenagers. "This guy was having a good time. Everyone have a look before class is over."

Some weeks later, my group was the one to make an exciting discovery. We identified Blanche's gallbladder, a small organ found in the upper right abdomen, and observed that its surface was irregular, bulging, and studded with bumps.

"Blanche has gallstones!" Alex exclaimed.

"Who has gallstones?" the professor asked, heading our way.

"Our cadaver goes by Blanche," Alex replied matter-of-factly as he affectionately patted her sallow hand. The professor was well-acquainted with Alex's sense of humor and shook his head with a smile.

"What are the four risk factors for cholecystitis?" he asked the rest of us.

"Fat, female, forty, and fertile," I droned along with my

groupmates as if reciting a Gregorian chant. I knew the 4Fs as if they were the names of my four children. Gallstones (cholelithiasis) and gallbladder inflammation (cholecystitis) are more common in women (Female) who are overweight or obese (Fat), middle-aged (Forty), and pregnant or of childbearing age (Fertile). Professors and classmates always shared unsolicited acronyms and mnemonics to help us remember groups of medical facts or terms: MUDPILES for causes of anion gap metabolic acidosis, Rad Techs Drink Cold Beer for the root subdivisions of the brachial plexus. Words and language have always affected me in a certain way, and I was more likely to remember only the silly saying and not what it stood for. The 4Fs, however, came up time and time again in classes and on tests until they became ingrained in my brain. According to our professors, we should immediately conjure up this checklist of risk factors if a female patient said she had right upper abdominal pain, nausea, and vomiting after eating.

"This woman still has her gallbladder, so the gallstones probably weren't giving her any problems," the professor told us as Alex mouthed 'Blanche' at me. "If she had acute cholecystitis, they wouldn't waste any time doing surgery. Go ahead, Alex, open it up."

Alex made a small slit in Blanche's gallbladder with a scalpel and tiny, coarse, greenish-black stones emerged. Some students moved closer, wide-eyed as if beholding the unlocking of a centuries-old treasure chest. I, on the other hand, willed myself not to escape to the hallway for fresh air. I thought formaldehyde had already obliterated my sense of smell, but a stench even more fetid escaped from the dissected gallbladder. One of my classmates, who was pregnant, gagged involuntarily and stepped back from the table.

Alex glanced at her growing belly.

"I just had a brilliant idea," he announced, his eyes glinting. "Blanche's gallstones would be perfect for a baby rattle. It'll be your most memorable baby shower gift ever."

"That's disgusting, Alex," she retorted with an eye roll.

A few months later, my lab group met to study for the final exam. Our professors would place small pins in cadavers and ask us to "identify this structure," "tell us which nerve innervates this structure," or "tell us which blood vessel lies next to this structure." Many of the body parts would be isolated from the rest of the cadaver, so we would need to orient ourselves and figure out what area we were looking at.

Alex burst into the lab ten minutes late, breathing hard.

"You guys will not believe what happened," he said anxiously as we regarded him with concern. "My cat was making a ton of noise in the closet today and wouldn't knock it off. I finally went in there to make her stop, and when I opened the door, a bunch of Blanche's gallstones rolled out. Oh my god, you guys. It smelled HORRIBLE." We stared at Alex in disbelief, then busted out laughing.

"You actually took those home?" I asked. I couldn't think of a more disgusting place than anatomy lab, especially one I returned to of my own free will. I shuddered at the thought of part of it coming home with me. If it were socially acceptable to strip down and shower in the lab, I would.

"Yeah, I took them home because I was going to make Lauren a baby rattle. But I just threw them in the closet and forgot about them until the cat discovered them." Alex glanced at Lauren's still-pregnant belly.

"Technically, I guess it's not too late to make the rattle, huh? She hasn't had the baby yet."

That glorious day when I walked out of anatomy lab for the last time, I thought to myself how things had come full circle. In high school, the Meyers-Briggs personality test that all the seniors took recommended a funeral director as my top career choice based on my ESFJ personality type (Extroverted, Sensing, Feeling, Judging). Broadly characterized as "The Provider,"

ESFJs are allegedly energized when spending time around other people, sensitive to their needs, and fulfilled by taking care of them. They are driven by feelings and values when making decisions, and they need organization and structure to thrive. This was a fairly accurate description of me, but funeral director had to be the vocation most *unlike* me. I was repulsed by death in any form and went to great lengths to avoid thinking or talking about it. Death was supposed to be a natural end that inevitably arrived for everyone. The only dead things I had ever seen, though, were animals that had been mangled by cars, neglected as pets, or killed for food and strung up in a window display. People, not nature, had caused death in all those circumstances. I had not personally known anyone who had died. Thus, death was unnatural, gruesome, something to be feared and avoided. I had even hated dissecting animals in high school biology because I felt like I was hurting innocent creatures. The frog, cow eye, sheep heart, fetal cat, pig . . . these animals all could have lived in harmony on Old MacDonald's farm, but instead were condemned to a formaldehyde-soaked bucket so that kids—most of whom wouldn't need biology, much less anatomy, at their future jobs—could tear their innards out and dangle them in front of each other like grotesque worms. Spending every day talking about death, walking among corpses, seeing dead people lying in coffins with faces covered in makeup . . . none of it was me.

Yet somehow, I had inadvertently managed to spend hours and hours with dead bodies in Gross Anatomy lab, and had accumulated more exposure to a single dead person than a funeral director would. I had inspected and explored every raw, reeking inch. I had seen corpses whose faces had no makeup, and who were not clothed in their Sunday best or arranged to look like they were simply sleeping. The irony. I took this as evidence that I had reached the point of no return. I wasn't going to stop at anything to become a PA.

CHILD'S PLAY

Twenty-one. The age when I could legally drink and, I was told, it was time to choose a career. With college graduation just months away, I had only a slightly less hazy idea of what I wanted to do with my life than I did as a freshman. I had followed a pre-health track; perhaps my empathetic nature, interpersonal skills, and penchant for organization might make me good at medicine. After all, I was "the provider."

If I was honest with myself, science never came easily to me. My parents, both medical physicists from China, could not hide their disbelief and disappointment when I barely scraped by in a college intro to physics class. I struggled with a degree of vacillation that I never witnessed in my pre-med classmates. Their clear visions of the path to becoming doctors and their cutthroat attitudes of wanting to be the best of the best escaped me. Once, I overhead one of them arguing passionately with our chemistry professor about a grade on an exam—a 95% versus a 98%, which she thought she should have received. Not once had I cared about a high A versus a slightly less-than-high A; I was content with simply scoring above the class average. I wasn't convinced that being "the best" would guarantee happiness, the thing I wanted most in life. The pride and fleeting pleasure of achievement or recognition simply could not compare to the joy I felt when I could be myself around people, when I didn't have the pressure of results, when I experienced new things and they challenged my existing beliefs. Since I was a child, my parents had always encouraged me to follow my dreams, so long as they didn't lead me to become a starving artist. As they watched me try to figure out my future, they made it clear that a job in liberal arts or a gap year after college was the precise path to the starving artist life. Science it was, then.

My roommate's mother, a physician, ultimately introduced the PA idea to me one night over dinner. I'd never heard of the profession, which came about in the '60s to address a nationwide need for primary care physicians. More doctors were gravitating towards specialties like otolaryngology, dermatology, and ophthalmology, and even those who chose primary care could not ease the shortage quickly enough because medical training took up to twelve years. PAs emerged to fill the gap. After two to two-and-a-half years of master's level education, they entered the workforce as "midlevel" clinicians. While they had designated supervising physicians they could consult for questions or assistance, PAs saw patients independently rather than assist physicians as their professional title suggested. They comprised a team that included doctors, nurses, technicians, and other medical staff.

My underdeveloped 21-year-old brain liked the sound of this PA life: shorter schooling and on-the-job training instead of a four-year medical residency meant I could be working and saving lives by age twenty-four, caring for people who would otherwise wait months or years to see a doctor. The blood, sweat, and tears that went into my hard-won science degree would not be for nothing. I was also attracted to the prospects of financial independence and work-life balance. Most PAs made six figures, which would be the equivalent of winning the lottery after the minimum-wage jobs I'd had in college ("Mom and I are not your bank," Dad reminded me as

I seriously contemplated whether I should eat only cereal for a week or splurge on a $10 Chipotle burrito). By the time I was thirty, the age at which most of my pre-med classmates would complete residency and start their first jobs, I might have paid off most of my school loans and even have a family. Physicians often sacrificed personal relationships or postponed having children due to the staggering strain of residency. Finally, PAs' general medicine education, with options to specialize and even change specialties, appealed to me. I couldn't even make this initial career selection, much less imagine committing to a specialty versus primary care for the rest of my life like I would if I went to med school. Now, indecisive me had the flexibility and freedom to choose! This occupation seemed to have everything I valued.

I felt pressured for time, however; some PA school application deadlines had already passed. Meanwhile, my classmates had already accepted high-paying jobs at Deloitte, Schlumberger, and Memorial Hermann. I shadowed an experienced and charismatic dermatology PA for one day, and then trekked across campus to the small, white, single-story O'Connor House at Rice University (now Huff House) for career counseling services.

The friendly counselor for biology majors confirmed that I had met all the requirements to graduate with a degree. I excitedly shared my goal of PA school and asked if she could recommend a place for me to start my search. I don't remember the woman's face or name, but I will forever remember the way she laughed after I laid out my dream before her.

"Emily, PA school is child's play," she said with a wave of her hand, like the prospect was an annoying gnat. "What do you really want to do?" She folded her hands, smiled, and waited expectantly, like I must have accidentally misspoken, and I flashed back momentarily to the Meyers-Briggs personality test in high school that had spit out "funeral director" as my future job. The tables had turned; this time, the counselor was the one laughing at my career idea. Her smile presently morphed into a look of concern that I appeared to be serious about my decision. She reached into a drawer and slid a handout across the desk to me.

"I want you to go home and read this. No one from Rice goes to PA school, only med school, and I know you're smart enough to take the MCAT. Come back if you have any questions, and let's get you signed up."

I glanced at the handout but didn't pick it up. I had survived a tough college curriculum, agonized over what I considered to be a momentous decision, humbly asked for advice, and was told my dream was juvenile.

"What if I'm still pretty sure I want to go to PA school?" I pressed.

The college counselor shook her head sympathetically.

"I think you would be making a mistake. You're smarter than that, Emily. If you're still set on it, though, I'm sure you can Google the names of some PA schools online."

The counseling session lasted fewer than ten minutes total. I thanked her politely and trudged back to my dorm room with the handout that she was convinced would bring me to my senses. Years later, on hard days at work, her words frequently crossed my mind. I wish I could go back and tell her that PA school, and being a PA, was nothing like she had described. It was grueling, unpredictable, sometimes a shitshow—but never child's play.

DIDACTIC YEAR: PHYSICAL EXAMINATION

It was in PA school that I touched a man's prostate for the first time. Trained and paid to behave like real patients, standardized patients provided feedback to help PA and medical students improve our history-taking and physical examination skills. I remember repeatedly wondering that day: *who would willingly allow a bunch of twenty-somethings who don't know what they're doing to stick their fingers in his anus? Did he do this annually for every PA school class?* Somehow, it had never occurred to me that prostate exams were part of PA school. I guess I just imagined I would be splinting broken bones, tormenting children with tongue depressors, and doing magic with a stethoscope before impressively arriving at diagnoses of rare conditions. In any event, I never expected my first prostate exam to be on such a willing participant.

I glanced at some of my classmates; it was hard to say what they were thinking. They ranged in age from twenties to forties, some were engaged or married, and they all had different life experiences, sexual orientations, religious beliefs, and personal values. Maybe they had never seen a naked man, thought the standardized patient was in it for sexual gratification, or felt that it was wrong to touch an anus that wasn't their significant other's or of the same or different gender.

As I stood in line, one of my classmates whispered, "I hope they're paying him a lot for this."

"You couldn't pay me enough," I muttered in reply.

"What if he's just a volunteer?" another classmate quipped.

Fortunately, Baylor had been merciful enough not to start the Physical Examination course with this unforgettable experience. All of us had begun the class unsuspectingly, using Gross Anatomy as a blueprint to methodically examine every organ system for health or disease. Our predecessors had somehow determined a myriad of methods to tell us what was happening internally, and we were each assigned a classmate of the same gender to practice on. The sequence of exam steps for nearly every body part was the same: inspect (visualize), auscultate (listen with a stethoscope), percuss (use finger pads to tap on the skin), and palpate (press lightly or firmly with the hand). In the early days of the class, we'd go straight to auscultating or palpating. We'd feel for lymph nodes around the face and jawline, asking our partners if there was any tenderness, only for the professor to call a time-out and remind us to stop and look before ever laying a finger on the patient. Observe both sides of the face first to see if they are symmetrical. Are any areas red or swollen compared to the other side? It was a long time before we were able to ignore the natural inclination to touch the patient as the first step in our assessments. *Inspect, auscultate, percuss, palpate.*

Physical Examination soon forced us out of our comfort zones in other ways, too. The professor emphasized that we couldn't hone our skills without practicing in a realistic environment: examining the heart, lungs, abdomen, etc. involves direct skin contact. As instructed, we all showed up to class wearing athletic shorts and T-shirts. Avoiding eye contact with one another, we reluctantly removed our shirts, leaving the men bare-chested and the women in sports bras. We crossed our arms or huddled behind the long lecture tables like shy, pubescent adolescents. As the cold A/C blasted from a vent overhead, a classmate whispered under her breath and asked if her nipples were showing through her bra because she was getting goosebumps.

Just as I would one day ask patients, I asked my partner if she was okay with me examining an area before I uncovered it to start inspecting and auscultating. I learned to preemptively state what I was about to do next, especially if it involved touching the skin, so the patient could anticipate it and the encounter would feel less invasive. By the end of the semester, awkwardness and embarrassment had passed. We were all used to seeing each other in various states of undress and had long since branched out from our assigned partners to practicing on all our other classmates, especially if someone's pulses were more prominent than normal or someone else's lung sounds were wheezy. Even I got to contribute during one session. The reflexes in my knees and feet were exaggerated compared to a "normal" person's, and the class gathered round as the professor and different students drummed on my kneecaps with reflex hammers like they were playing a xylophone. When they found the correct spot on the tendon, my leg would involuntarily kick out to their delight, and the area would buzz and tingle like I had hit my funny bone again and again. The professor then repositioned my leg on the table to demonstrate how to check for a blood clot. I was on full display, with forty pairs of eyes staring at me in my sports bra.

Without worrying about appearances, we were able to focus on what was normal, what was abnormal, and different physical maneuvers we could use to either rule in or rule out a likely diagnosis. Our partly naked bodies weren't provocative or sexual; they were simply road maps if we knew how to read them. The final test was a timed, comprehensive, head-to-toe physical exam on our partner utilizing all the techniques we had learned. The professor asked questions throughout about how to interpret the findings, and we verbally described every action as we performed it: "I'm checking that the trachea is midline and mobile. I'm palpating for the liver edge to feel for enlargement or irregularity." Physical Examination helped us understand and expect that discomfort was a natural part of learning and growing into our roles as PAs.

Nevertheless, any profound insight momentarily went out the window as I dragged my feet towards the testicles that drooped between the standardized patient's hairy legs and the rectum that several gloved fingers coated in lube had already prodded. He stood with his back to us in a loosely tied hospital gown, which fell open to expose his backside each time he bent over the table before him. The man was exceedingly tolerant; if students did not feel his prostate on the first attempt, he let them try again so they could learn proper technique. We were supposed to "gently" place a finger against the anus to encourage the muscle to relax before palpating. I nearly gagged and closed my eyes when I inserted my finger. It took everything in me not to recoil.

"That wasn't too bad," the standardized patient said encouragingly as he straightened up and faced me. "Remember to ask the patient to bear down so you can feel the sphincter. You did a good job."

I was positively baffled by how this man seemed so nonchalant, like we were just looking into his ears or something. A small part of me wondered if my classmates were right, that he was getting some kind of sexual gratification from this exercise. What he couldn't tell me was that, a few years later, patients would specifically request me rather than the male clinicians for their prostate exams because my fingers were smaller, and they assumed it would be less uncomfortable. Ironically, small fingers must reach farther to make contact with the intended target.

I mumbled a thank you to the standardized patient and removed my glove (inside out, as I had been taught, so as not to contaminate anything else with body fluids) like it was a used condom. *What did I get myself into?*

DIDACTIC YEAR:

CULTURAL (IN)COMPETENCY

Arnold was our professor for Cultural Competency, a course where we became familiar with the concepts of implicit bias and respectful care for patients from different backgrounds. Among the first graduating classes of PAs in the United States, Arnold was knowledgeable, charismatic, and took his responsibility of teaching the next generation of PAs very seriously. His anecdotes were always entertaining, and I was curious as to what he'd share in the day's lecture, entitled "Traditions: Asian Americans," as an older white gentleman. He didn't disappoint.

"Merchants sold things to others," Arnold read off a slide which was meant to enlighten us about Asian history. Alex (the one who nabbed the gallstones) gave me a meaningful look, then double-underlined this statement on his printout.

"Sold things to others," he repeated solemnly, just low enough so that Arnold couldn't hear him. "Every day, I learn something new." I tried to keep a straight face. Then I heard Arnold describe bowing to a physician every time they passed each other in the hospital cafeteria, addressing the latter by his formal title because he was Japanese. Japanese people give a "long, low bow" and never use first names to address each other, Arnold explained. The physician usually returned a quick bow or nod, but Arnold insisted that it would be deeper if the recipient was of higher standing because bowing signified respect. We snorted and shook our heads as he demonstrated small versus deep bows, looking as out of place as a white actor portraying a person of color in a movie.

Next, Arnold recounted sharing his love of sushi with Chinese patients to build rapport (sushi, by the way, is part of Japanese cuisine). I watched with a mixture of amusement and incredulousness as he indicated a picture of a few pieces of sushi on the screen with his laser pointer. You could bow slightly to Chinese and Chinese American patients when you greeted them if you wished, Arnold said, although a handshake was also acceptable. I kept my eyes straight ahead even as I could see Alex trembling with laughter beside me. He nudged me and pointed to a couple of students in front of us who sat with rapt attention, diligently scribbling notes.

"What are they writing?" he mouthed at me.

Finally, Arnold spoke about playing pool with Mexican friends (last time I checked, Mexicans are not Asian). They called him *gringo*, an affectionate nickname that made him part of the group despite their different native languages.

A wave of comments ensued as we filed out of the lecture hall.

"That Japanese doctor bowed back and was probably wondering, 'Why is this white man bowing at me?'" one classmate guffawed.

"What I'm worried about is what notes they were taking," another replied, referring to the students who asked serious questions and didn't appear to find the presentation or the associated gestures absurd. "'Small bows to Chinese patients and deep bows to Japanese ones?'"

Indeed, all our professor had taught us was stereotypes that different Asian ethnic groups face. He did not acknowledge the often stark contrast in beliefs and practices between people who live in Asia and people of Asian descent who grow up and live in America. I had certainly never bowed at anyone, nor observed any of the other so-called traditions Arnold spoke of. None of the Asians I knew did, either, and

I found it comical, outrageous even, that anyone believed this was how they behaved. How naïve of me! I was blissfully unaware of how my physical appearance would influence the way patients viewed me. Soon, we'd be putting our medical knowledge and skills into practice, which felt like constantly treading water to try to learn everything. In addition, I would field questions and comments from patients about my ethnicity during nearly every clinical rotation. The truth was, I was even more out of touch than Arnold about what it meant to be Asian American. I had no concept of my identity and was in for quite the rude awakening.

WAIT...I'M ASIAN?

After the White Coat Ceremony, our clinical rotations began for internal medicine, pediatrics, emergency medicine, community medicine, obstetrics and gynecology, and electives. They lasted four to eight weeks each, and we were assigned to a team with a preceptor and medical students, interns, and residents from other programs. Clinical Year was our first dive into direct patient care, a taste of what the rest of our career would be like. I introduced myself to each patient as a PA student and started awkwardly asking questions and examining them so I could report the conclusions to my attending physician.

On my first day on the inpatient internal medicine ward at Houston VA Hospital, an elderly patient caught sight of me and gasped sharply before tossing the bedsheet over his head. Curiously, I came closer and tugged on the corner, but he only snatched it tighter.

"Mr. Lehman, I'm the physician assistant student, Emily," I said, bemused. I heard heavy breathing, and then the sheet stirred slightly as Mr. Lehman's eyes appeared over its edge.

"Are you playing hide and seek?" I joked. He didn't laugh.

"You remind me of the girls when I was in Vietnam," he said finally, his voice muffled.

"Well, we're not in Vietnam right now, and I'm not Vietnamese," I said lamely, unsure how to respond. "I'm just here to see how you're doing and to get you feeling better. Can we go over your medications?"

I did not ask Mr. Lehman which Vietnamese girls I reminded him of, but I knew that many veterans who witness war or death have post-traumatic stress disorder. Reminders of those experiences are distressing and can bring back not only unwanted emotions but also intense physical reactions. Mr. Lehman might have been referring to innocent women and girls who were killed when he fought in Vietnam. He might have been referring to women he'd had sex with there. Or perhaps, he was remembering the women who volunteered as nurses during the war. In any event, the association was clearly negative. I spent the next ten minutes coaxing Mr. Lehman out of the sheets and encouraging him to talk so that we could discuss his treatment. He continued to regard me with suspicion throughout the entire exchange, and it was only after repeated visits over the following days that he eventually accepted that this particular Asian was harmless.

Although it was eye-opening, I didn't feel strongly about the situation; Houston is the fourth biggest city in the United States and diverse—I was hardly the only Asian there. Mr. Lehman's perception of me must just be a coincidence because untold ghosts haunted him as a veteran. He had served our country, and I was here to serve him.

Gradually, though, I started to feel like my white coat was embroidered with *Hi, I'm Asian!* As I scarfed down my lunch outside the hospital's main entrance one day, a patient walked by and remarked, "Is there a Chinatown nearby? That looks like the flan that you can only find in Oriental stores." It was pumpkin pie I had bought at Target.

Later that week, my classmate, Ray, and I chatted outside after our shift with our scrubs and stethoscopes still on. We were exhausted. We had both been involved in complex patient cases where it seemed like the hospital system had ground to a halt and prevented us from helping. The "urgent" MRIs and CTs we had ordered took days before available staff and space on the schedule allowed the patient to be transported to the imaging department, and then it took several more days before the images and reports returned from the radiologists. We'd always just expected that once we formulated a plan and ordered the appropriate tests, the results would guide us smoothly to the answer so we could neatly wrap up patients' problems. Instead, we found ourselves mired in the red tape of health insurance company requirements, hospital administration restrictions, and patient financial limitations.

"Next week will be better," Ray said, giving me a hug. "I'll see you Monday."

As we said goodbye and I turned to walk to my car, a man approached me. He appeared to be lost. Ray stuck around protectively, since it was getting dark and we were the only ones in the parking lot.

"Can we help you, sir?" Ray asked.

"I was just going to my car, but then I saw y'all and had to tell you," the man said excitedly. "This is straight out of *Grey's Anatomy*. Two good-looking doctors talking, an Asian and a redhead."

We watched in silence as he walked away, laughing to himself. Then Ray winked at me.

"If you weren't here, I'd probably just be some redhead standing on the curb. Now I'm McSteamy."

Some patients didn't hesitate at all to jump right in and start speaking to me in Chinese. Newsflash: I speak English. When I accompanied my attending, Dr. Lindsey, to a procedure one morning, she pulled me aside and said, "Just giving you a heads-up: this patient will probably speak to you in another language. She considers herself very cultured and open-minded, and I've seen her do it to anyone of a different background than her."

I shrugged. "Okay."

The patient was a pleasant woman and paid hardly any attention to me during the appointment. She chatted casually with Dr. Lindsey, and I quickly forgot about Dr. Lindsey's comment. When we turned to leave, the patient suddenly called out, "Xie xie" ("thank you" in Chinese) with a nearly incomprehensible accent. I paused, knowing full well that the statement was intended for me, and stole a glance at Dr. Lindsey. She looked simply tickled and mouthed, "See?"

"You're welcome," I said stiffly in English, feeling obliged to respond but desperate for the conversation to be over.

"C'mon! You *are* fluent in Chinese, aren't you?" the patient pressed.

"No."

"Can you read and write it?"

"Nope."

In fact, I'd stammer out a few broken, grammatically incorrect Chinese sentences and phrases once every few years as my parents looked on, wondering where all those years of Chinese school went.

Chinese schools are fairly common in the United States. Asian Americans learn to read and write Chinese, try traditional activities such as dance and martial arts, and practice public speaking. I attended Chinese school starting in kindergarten but, as a result of disuse, had long since forgotten how to read, write, and speak Mandarin. I also had zero experience with medical Chinese and saw the language as part of my parents' culture, not mine.

On another occasion, a Hispanic/Latinx patient I'd only seen in passing got on the elevator with me.

"What floor?" I asked him politely.

"Di bah ceng" ("the eighth floor" in Chinese).

I gave a small, fake laugh as I turned away to press the elevator button.

"You understood what I was saying!" the patient said behind me, sounding pleased. "My wife is learning Chinese, so I'm picking up some, too."

"Your Chinese is better than mine," I told him, and smiled graciously although I really didn't feel like repeatedly having variations of this conversation.

We rode the rest of the way to the eighth floor in silence. As the doors opened and he stepped out, the patient turned to me and started trying to say "have a good day" in Chinese. He was having trouble coming up with one of the words when the doors started closing.

As I stood alone in that elevator, simultaneously confused and exasperated by this new thing where people felt the need to speak to me in Chinese or otherwise reference my ethnicity, the concept of cultural competency finally sank in. It was a disconcerting and alienating feeling when people made assumptions about me based on my appearance. I vowed then and there never to be the one to make a patient feel the same way.

CLINICAL YEAR: OB/GYN

My OB/GYN rotation took place at a busy clinic just outside of Houston. On my second day, I followed the OB into her office where a woman and a little girl, her niece, waited for their consultation. I thought the aunt was the patient, but quickly realized my mistake when Dr. Larson opened the manila folder containing the patient's chart. The photo was of the little girl.

"Hi Mia, your aunt tells me you had sex with a boy at school," Dr. Larson said in a slightly questioning tone.

Mia didn't say anything. She pressed methodically with her thumb along the row of a push pop bubble fidget toy that all the kids seemed to have these days. Her date of birth indicated that she was nine, but she looked barely older than five. She wore a powder blue Gap T-shirt and Crocs studded with shoe charms.

"Mia, put that away and talk to the doctor," her aunt said gently.

Dr. Larson smiled encouragingly and tried again. "Mia, do you know his name?"

Mia paused for a long time before saying no in a tiny voice. Her aunt clarified that she believed Mia did know the boy's name but didn't want her aunt or her parents to know.

"Did the boy touch you when you didn't want to, or make you have sex with him?" Dr. Larson continued.

"No, I wanted to," Mia said calmly, her face expressionless.

"And did he put anything on his penis before you had sex, like a condom?"

"No."

I felt strange, like I had intruded upon a very private conversation. I didn't even know what a condom was when I was nine years old, much less how to have sex, and I studied Mia's soft brown eyes with a mixture of pity and sympathy. She was so young to have to go through this interrogation.

Dr. Larson spoke again. "What grade are you in, Mia?"

"Third grade."

"Have you ever had sex with anyone else?"

"No. Just the boy at school."

"Okay. When was the last time you had your period?"

"I dunno."

"I think it was three months ago," the aunt volunteered. "She just started them this year; she doesn't have bleeding every month yet."

"That's very normal. Mia, after a girl has a period, she can get pregnant anytime if she has sex with a boy, even if it's just once. Do you understand what that means?"

"Yeah."

Dr. Larson raised one eyebrow slightly, but her tone remained even. "Today we did a test, and you are pregnant. That means there is a baby inside of you right now." Dr. Larson tilted her chin to catch Mia's eye, and I watched with bated breath to see if Mia registered what the doctor was saying. She stared, still expressionless, her Crocs dangling above the floor because her legs couldn't reach the ground. Her aunt, meanwhile, had the exact opposite reaction and squeezed Mia into an ebullient hug.

"Oh, Mia! You are going to be a mother!" She stroked Mia's hair and murmured something in Spanish to her. Dr. Larson looked surprised.

"In our culture, being able to have children is very important for women," the aunt explained, turning to us. She was delighted that Mia was fertile and added with a wink, "Even if it is a little sooner than we expected."

Dr. Larson didn't return her smile. I marveled at the way she proceeded to counsel the aunt with both cultural respect and concern for the effects of preteen pregnancy on school, social life, Mia's body, and her future goals. Abortion was still legal in Texas at the time, and when Dr. Larson delicately broached the subject, the aunt firmly refused and maintained that Mia's parents would do the same. Dr. Larson appeared weary but agreed to a follow-up with Mia, her parents, and her aunt.

My head was spinning as Dr. Larson and I watched them leave. Nine years old, third grade, and ... a mother. Should we be reporting this to someone?

As if she had read my mind, Dr. Larson told me solemnly, "We see things like this a lot, unfortunately. In Texas, the age of consent is seventeen. But since the boy Mia had sex with is the same age as her and isn't a sex offender, he probably won't be charged with anything. The sad thing is, Mia's not even the youngest mother who's come to see me. The problem isn't teenage pregnancy anymore—it's preteen pregnancy." And with that, she closed Mia's chart and strode out of the room. On to the next one.

My OB/GYN rotation also taught me never to assume a woman was too old to get pregnant. A patient was referred to our clinic after she noticed pain and swelling in her abdomen and weight gain. She went to her primary care provider (PCP) because she thought she had a tumor, but a few quick tests told a different story.

As Dr. Larson and I headed to the exam room, the nurse pulled us aside.

"Ms. George wouldn't let me check her blood pressure or temperature, and she tore the exam paper off the table. She was yelling that this is such BS, that her kids are grown and it's a tumor and she needs to see an oncologist."

Dr. Larson gave me a meaningful look that said *brace yourself*. When we opened the door, shredded exam paper covered the floor like bits of wrapping paper on Christmas morning. The pen holder and a few instruments were knocked out of place, and a glowering woman stood in the middle of the room with her hands folded across her chest.

"Hello, I'm Dr. Larson," my attending said, graciously extending her hand and ignoring the mess.

"Jesus Christ, how many times do I have to tell you people—I have a tumor!" Ms. George shrieked, refusing to uncross her arms.

"Your PCP ran some tests, and he doesn't think you have a tumor," Dr. Larson replied patiently, sitting down. "He sent you here because your pregnancy test was positive, so we're going to use ultrasound today to take a look. It won't hurt; it feels kind of like a tampon."

Ms. George rolled her eyes and begrudgingly lay down for the ultrasound, continuing to mutter about how she was fifty-six years old, how her children were already grown, and how this was the biggest waste of time and money because she really needed to be seeing a cancer doctor. After a few minutes, Dr. Larson turned the ultrasound screen so that both Ms. George and I could see it, while maintaining firm pressure with the ultrasound probe.

"Ms. George, you are in fact pregnant. The good news is that it's in the right spot. We wanted to make sure you didn't have an ectopic pregnancy, where the fertilized egg grows inside the fallopian tube. That's a surgical emergency."

"I'm pregnant?! This is crazy! How can you be sure it's a baby and not cancer?"

"You see this thing that's moving right here? That's the baby's heart."

Ms. George stared in disbelief at the valves wiggling on the computer screen.

"Oh my god, this is insane. I'm too old for this! How is this possible?"

"A woman can get pregnant if she doesn't use protection every time she has sex," Dr. Larson replied bluntly, without a smile. I had to bite my lip at her direct response to Ms. George's rhetorical question, and, as the latter glared daggers, I busied myself with picking up the Christmas wrapping paper. When she finally calmed down, Ms. George seemed torn about how to proceed with the pregnancy. She quietly received the contact information for a maternal-fetal medicine specialist, since older women are at higher risk of pregnancy complications, as well as for a clinician who performed abortions because Dr. Larson did not provide that particular service. I never knew which path Ms. George ultimately took, since I was only at the clinic for four weeks.

While routine prenatal visits, well-woman exams, birth control consultations, and vaginal discharge evaluations comprised the majority of clinic appointments, deliveries always took precedence. Often, as Dr. Larson moved through her daily roster of patients, her cell phone would suddenly blare a distinct ringtone, signaling us to drop whatever we were doing, let the patient know we were off to deliver a baby, and jump into Dr. Larson's convertible to head to the delivery hospital. Dr. Larson really had two jobs as an OB/GYN, and she switched back and forth between them like an ambidextrous baseball batter.

She never put her seatbelt on or locked the car doors. Putting on a seatbelt, she said, was time wasted because every second counted during delivery. Consequently, the incessant dinging of the seatbelt alert accompanied us for the entire three- to five-minute exhilarating ride to the hospital. I smelled rubber burning as Dr. Larson screeched out of her reserved clinic parking spot onto the feeder road and tore across five lanes of Texas highway to the hospital like she was in a real-life version of Mario Kart, liable at any moment to spin out on a pesky banana peel, which would end in our fiery deaths. Dr. Larson never once hit the brake until we reached the labor and delivery doors. Sometimes, she even left the car running, parked horizontally across the three reserved spots for OBs, and entrusted me with straightening the car out before meeting her on the labor and delivery unit. I thought about how ironic it would be if we died in a car accident on our way to bring life into the world.

This was how I came to see a live birth for the first time in my life, and dozens more within the coming weeks. At the first delivery I attended, I didn't see the baby come out or anything like that. When we entered the room, the mother was drenched in sweat, and her hair and hospital gown were glued to her skin. She was screaming at the father, who sat on a bench about ten feet from her bed looking like he was about to hurl. His face was a milky shade of green, and he wasn't making eye contact with anyone.

"GET. OVER. HERE!" the mother screamed in Spanish, each word more laborious than the last as she cried out with anger and pain. The father remained glued to his spot like a horrified statue.

Dr. Larson, meanwhile, had assumed her position below the mother's legs and busied herself with various instruments. She announced to the room that the baby was crowning, meaning that the top of its head was visible, and commanded the mother to push. As the mother bellowed with her first push, the father chose that moment to bolt out of the room, presumably to find a toilet to throw up in. Dr. Larson and the L&D nurses all talked loudly at the foot of the bed, where I stood as well. None of them looked at the mother's face, which was the picture of abject misery.

Something happened inside me that I can't explain since I'd never met the mother or father before, nor experienced childbirth. I rushed to the head of the bed, grabbed the mother's hand, and pushed the sweat-soaked strands of hair out of her face. She was in so much agony and there were so many people around her legs that I don't think she even noticed me. Using my best conversational Spanish, I encouraged her as she pushed her first baby out to life and we heard, with joy and relief, its cute little cry. Afterward, the mother slumped back on the pillow and sobbed as the nurse cut the umbilical cord. Dr. Larson usually let the father do the honors, but he still hadn't returned.

As the mother held her baby in her arms for the first time, she looked at me and quietly said in English, "Thank you." We didn't know each other's names, and we would never see each other again.

CLINICAL YEAR:
PIMPIN' AIN'T EASY

No, not *that* kind of pimping. For PA and medical students, we universally knew that "pimping" referred to the centuries-old practice in which an attending physician put us on the spot in front of the medical team and asked rapid-fire clinical questions. Attendings could pimp us at any time, without warning, and if we didn't know the answer, they moved on to someone else and posed the same question. If we answered incorrectly, there were two possible outcomes: they either ignored us or reamed us like we were the scum of the earth. Nor could we congratulate ourselves if we got the answers right; attendings often asked additional questions until they eventually stumped us. Pimping allegedly came into existence to help students think quickly on their feet, move beyond rote memorization to sound clinical reasoning, and recognize the necessity of constant learning and preparation. Pimping was our unavoidable inauguration into Clinical Year, and, just as Ice-T said, pimpin' ain't easy.

Once during my general surgery rotation, a medical student and I stood on opposite sides of an unconscious patient in the operating room. After we had stretched the incision site wide with retractors, the attending pointed to an organ and asked the medical student which organ was next to it and which blood vessel supplied it. The medical student stammered out a wrong answer uncertainly and was promptly told, "Get out of my sight."

My head was next on the chopping block. I summoned

the relevant anatomy, and a mixture of relief and guilt washed over me. Both the medical student and I passed anatomy class to advance to this clinical rotation. Had he been less flustered, he would undoubtedly have arrived at the correct answer. Now, he was beating himself up in the hallway. We had all been there, thinking ourselves the stupidest human being in the world and doubting whether we could really do this kind of work. Pimping does that to a person.

I was pimped plenty more times on clinicals. My emergency medicine attending, a middle-aged man of formidable stature who seemingly never smiled, once instructed me to take a patient's history in front of their family and the medical team. The patient, a young man who looked quite uncomfortable in the hospital bed, told me he had abdominal pain, and I asked the standard questions I'd been trained on: Where's the pain? How long has it been going on? What makes the pain better or worse? Then I proceeded to a review of systems, which involved learning about any relevant symptoms from other organ systems that might help establish a diagnosis for the abdominal pain.

I had scarcely started when the attending sharply interrupted to ask why my questions didn't follow any kind of logical order. The patient, his family, and everyone on the team stared at me, waiting for my answer.

"I asked about the gastrointestinal symptoms, so now I'm doing a review of systems," I said without a trace of attitude.

"Who taught you to do the review of systems that way?" the attending barked.

"School."

"Well school got it wrong. Do it from head to toe so you don't miss anything."

I apologized and changed tactics as instructed for the remainder of the history.

"You're dismissed for the day," the attending said when I was finished, with no word as to whether the second attempt had been better. I thanked the patient and his family, and my team watched silently as I walked away. The fact that everyone knew I was a student and still in training didn't comfort me in the slightest.

Over the next few weeks, I practiced the same method of history-taking and the attending did not interrupt me again, so I figured I was getting the hang of it. Others did not get the same treatment. On one occasion, he yelled at a medical student, "Do they teach you guys *anything* in medical school?" and I watched sympathetically as her eyes welled up with tears.

At the end of each clinical rotation, the preceptor submits a performance evaluation and a letter grade to Baylor. I couldn't help but laugh at my emergency medicine attending's final snub at my PA program before we parted ways: "Emily responded well to my requirement that she see patients, interview, and present in a clear and logical fashion, rather than according to the template which she has been taught, which is illogical and counterproductive, and which encourages the practice of bad medicine." Although he was curt, uncompromising, and sometimes yelled at students like he wanted their blood, I almost grew fond of him. Unlike many attendings, who made it seem like their life goal was to break and publicly guillotine students for entertainment, he capitalized on teachable moments and dispensed tough love so we could become good PAs and physicians. I started to appreciate that attendings were once pimped themselves as students and residents, and were now responsible for shaping up the next generation of clinicians. Taking criticism too personally was self-destructive when we knew so little in the expansive world of modern medicine.

Pimping's other widely reported purpose was to establish and reinforce a pecking order in medicine: the attending was the all-knowing power, the fellow and residents his right-hand stewards, and the intern and medical/PA students the lowly pond scum. All of the above were present when the medical team rounded on patients, and anyone higher than me on the totem pole could pimp me.

As I finished up my patient notes one evening on my internal medicine rotation, the intern on my team received a page. Our patient who had surgery earlier in the week now had a fever.

"What could be causing her fever?" the intern asked me after he hung up the phone.

"An infection of the surgical site," I answered confidently.

"What else could cause it?"

"An infection somewhere else in the body?" I answered less confidently. He shot me a look like a kindergartener could give a better answer.

"Emily, that's a cop-out. What are the five possible causes of post-op fever? Don't you know the five Ws?"

I searched the darkest corners of my brain for this undoubtedly illuminating mnemonic; nothing emerged. The only five Ws I had ever heard of were *who, what, when, where, why*. As all PA students know when they get pimped, the answer is never *I don't know*, even if that's the case. Instead, we say, *I don't know, but I'll find out*. I dutifully consulted the pocket reference book in my short white coat pocket and recited it to the intern's satisfaction: Wound, Water, Wind, Walking, and Wonder drugs. As it turned out, "wind" was responsible for our patient's post-op fever—she had atelectasis, where part of the lung collapses. While acronyms and mnemonics would still continue to escape me, I never forgot the five Ws.

Perhaps that was pimping's other function: to engender humility and reframe our idealistic mindsets as students that it is ever possible to know it all or be the best. I understood that, at this moment, my place was as pond scum. Surprisingly, I didn't mind it all that much.

Clinical Year:
Emergency Medicine

I was simultaneously the most excited by and most terrified of my emergency medicine rotation, which would take place at Ben Taub Hospital, a Level I trauma center in Houston. Ben Taub was where people went after gunshot wounds, suicide attempts, gruesome accidents, and other critical, life-threatening conditions. I later learned that it was also the first point of contact for people with everyday concerns like colds or foot pain that would be better addressed by a PCP. Many who came to the ED had no health insurance, much less a PCP, and the Emergency Medical Treatment and Labor Act (EMTALA) required us to treat everyone, regardless of insurance status or ability to pay.

Unlike my previous rotations in internal medicine and OB/GYN, where I typically interviewed and examined patients as part of a team or observed my attending, I largely saw patients on my own in the ED. There was no orientation. I located my designated attending for the day and was off to see the next patient in his or her queue moments later. It didn't take long for me to understand that in emergency medicine, more than in any other specialty, the "chief complaint" was king. As the first line of every medical note, the chief complaint describes the reason the patient is seeking medical care. It is usually a brief sentence in his or her own words, but can also be summarized as a phrase or symptom. Chief complaints ranged from unassuming to mind-blowing, and at Ben Taub, I never knew which one it was going to be.

Chief Complaint: Rash

A page went off overhead one day: "Emily Zhu to ED Room 13. Emily Zhu to ED Room 13."

I had never heard my name over the ED's intercom before. I apologized to the patient I was evaluating and hurried toward Room 13 while a litany of worst-case scenarios made their way through my head. *Had I ordered the wrong test? Did a patient tell my attending that I got the story wrong? Did something bad happen to my patient? Oh shit, oh shit, oh shit.*

The attending and the patient both looked up as I stepped through the automatic doors into Room 13. The patient, a middle-aged woman in an oversized tie-dye T-shirt, reclined calmly on a hospital gurney and smiled. Nothing seemed amiss.

"Thanks for coming," the doctor said to me. "Grab a pair of gloves. Ms. Carson, this is our PA student."

"Hi Ms. Carson, I'm Emily," I introduced myself, slightly out of breath.

"Hi there, honey. I've got this rash, but I need a little assistance to show the doctor." Without warning, she pulled her shirt up. She wasn't wearing a bra.

"Help me lift this side, will ya? It's under here." Ms. Carson motioned to her pendulous right breast and grunted as I obediently lifted it. It was heavy as hell, damp underneath, and smelled musty.

The attending leaned over the gurney and shined his penlight on the red, angry rash from what seemed like every angle as I wondered whether it was possible to sprain my wrist under the crushing weight of a human breast. Ms. Carson appeared to have two perfectly functioning hands but made no effort to help lighten the load.

"Mm-hmm," the attending murmured, drawing my attention back to the rash. "I see some satellite lesions, so this is probably yeast. Emily, can you move it just a little higher?"

Chief Complaint: "I zipped up my dick"

3:48 a.m. I stifled a yawn as I looked at the computer screen. The minutes were crawling by during my third 7p-7a night shift out of six, and 4:00 a.m. was about the time each morning when drowsiness began to overtake me. After the switch from day shifts the previous week, the transition was brutal. The effects of my sleep deprivation, likely the equivalent of the legal blood alcohol limit, meant my clinical reasoning and decision-making took progressively longer as dawn approached. Earlier in the night, I had held out both hands in the shape of an L and a backward L, to confirm left and right before starting a procedure. I never did this to distinguish the two any other time in my life, not even when I learned them as a kid. This was the only thing my brain could produce to prevent a potentially dangerous mistake in its somnolent haze. The physical heaviness of sleep weighed on my body, and my mental acuity drifted away like a whisper in the wind.

The ED was relatively quiet that Saturday night; my patients were sleeping or waiting on test results. Then a young woman came in, her stilettos echoing across the tile floor as she approached the check-in desk. She was tall and slender, with a lacy minidress that showcased legs for days.

"Hi, my friend is outside and he needs some help," she told the triage nurse politely.

"What's the patient's name?" the nurse asked (unnecessarily loudly, I thought, since the waiting room was nearly empty).

"Nick."

"Last name?"

The young woman paused and stared like the nurse had

just asked her a complicated question. Just then, a young man appeared at the automatic doors and began limping toward us. The woman turned and called to him.

"Nick, what's your last name?"

"Capriano," he said, grimacing as he continued to take small, awkward steps.

"What are you coming in for, Mr. Capriano?" the nurse asked, her tone softer upon seeing the woman's stumbling companion. Nick and the woman exchanged glances before he mumbled a response. I couldn't hear his answer and, apparently, neither could the nurse.

"One more time? You zipped up . . . ?"

"My dick," Nick hissed through clenched teeth. He was turning red now. The young woman, meanwhile, looked like she could barely hold her laughter in. The nurse assigned the chart to my attending, and I filed into the triage room after them to take the initial history.

Within five minutes, I went from obtunded to wide awake. In a twist of events fitting for an episode of the TV show *Sex Sent Me to the ER*, 28-year-old Nick told me how he had gotten his penis stuck in his pants zipper. He had been on a first date earlier that night with the woman, Marissa (hence, she didn't even know his last name). They went to a popular Mexican restaurant in town and planned to go to a bar after to get another drink. Before they left, Nick made what was supposed to be a quick stop in the bathroom. He zipped up his jeans—and promptly caught his foreskin in his pants zipper.

"I was bent over the urinal trying not to pass out from the pain," Nick said bitterly. "I tried to pull the zipper back down, but that just made it worse. It felt like someone had cut my penis off."

"Something was off," Marissa added, looking at Nick

sympathetically. "The date was going really well, and it was weird when he came back from the bathroom sweaty and kind of disheveled. He seemed upset about something."

"That's when you told her what happened?" I asked Nick. He shook his head.

"I was trying not to let her see that I had my fly open, so I hunched over and made up some excuse that I had to go." The act of straightening up, though, had hit him with a new wave of pain and he cried out again. Alarmed, Marissa had begged him to tell her what was going on, and Nick finally admitted his embarrassing secret. She ordered him a shot and made him gulp it down to ease the pain before she drove him to the ED.

After I presented the case to my attending, he examined Nick and kept his face neutral even as he was probably cringing inside at the reddened skin trapped between the teeth and the slide of the zipper. We attempted to gently dislodge the zipper by pulling the skin in the opposite direction, but this was both unsuccessful and immensely painful. Next, I used trauma shears to cut off Nick's jeans so that only a thin piece of fabric with the zipper remained. We hoped that removing the weight of the jeans might be enough to free the skin, but again nothing happened. Applying lubricant and maneuvering Nick in all kinds of different positions did not work, either.

Finally, my attending stood next to Nick, whose junk was entirely exposed save for a strip of the attached zipper, and explained the only choice left: inject anesthesia into Nick's penis and "surgically" remove the zipper with pliers.

"No, no, I don't want to do any kind of injection," Nick protested, involuntarily covering his crotch with his hands. "Can you just rip the zipper off?"

"We can, but that's going to be very painful," the attending said, frowning.

"It's already painful. Please, just make it quick."

My attending sighed and nodded for me to assist him. Marissa grabbed both of Nick's hands and told him to keep looking straight at her the entire time. My attending secured the pliers around the zipper and *ZIP!*

Nick's scream could be heard throughout the emergency department bay. He lay on the hospital bed deflated and naked from the waist down as three pairs of eyes stared at his manhood. He looked too exhausted and relieved to even feel embarrassed. Marissa rubbed his shoulder sympathetically.

As far as memorable first dates go, I think that one takes the cake.

Chief Complaint: Burn

Another young man, a 25-year-old named Michael, came into the emergency department for a different unfortunate accident: second-degree burns on his hands after taking a pizza out of the oven without oven mitts. Michael's palms were puffy, shiny, red, and exquisitely tender to touch, and one was beginning to blister. I began gathering materials to dress the burns. After silently watching me work for a few minutes, Michael seemed to conclude that I was trustworthy and gave me the full story of how he got burned. He had awoken on the couch that morning to sunlight blinding him in his eyes and leaves blowing into his living room. His front door was standing wide open and his roommate, Scott, was passed out on the loveseat nearby.

"It was Scott's birthday last night and we partied pretty hard," Michael admitted. "I don't know why the door was open, but it didn't look like anyone had broken in or stolen anything."

As he walked over to close the door, something on the sidewalk caught his eye and he picked it up.

"I walk back inside, look up, and there's a hole in the ceiling with wires sticking out of it. Yep, it's my smoke detector. No idea why it was outside." Michael thought Scott might know something, so he asked him what happened.

"He told me that I grabbed a frozen pizza without even taking the plastic off and put it in the oven. The smoke alarm kept going off, and I got so annoyed that I ripped it off the ceiling, threw it out the door, and just went to sleep."

"Wow," I replied with a little laugh, thinking of how I'd had some similarly crazy nights when I was in college. I wasn't going to admit that, obviously.

"I noticed the red light for the oven was still on when I started picking up around the kitchen," Michael continued. "It smelled like burnt rubber when I opened the door, and heat and smoke blasted me in the face. I see this black, deformed blob on the rack and I'm like, 'Shit! The pizza!'"

And without thinking, Michael had reached in with both hands to pull out the pizza that had been cooking for over ten hours at 425 degrees.

The ED was always noisy and chaotic, and the list of patients on our computer screens never dwindled regardless of how many hours were left in our shifts. The goal was always to stabilize and discharge as quickly as possible; longer hospital stays increase the risk of infections and other complications, and freeing up beds meant fewer patients in hallways and holding areas. Our speed as students, of course, was constrained by inexperience and various other factors such as language barriers and unfamiliarity with the hospital and its electronic medical record (EMR) system. Our professors also cautioned us against rushing because we were dealing with lives and peoples' dignity.

According to the EMR, a young woman named Amber had arrived with a chief complaint of leg pain. She fidgeted uncomfortably on the hospital bed when I walked in, and once I pulled the curtain and asked her which leg was hurting, she admitted that she was too embarrassed to tell the check-in nurse the real reason she was here.

"Don't be embarrassed," I tried to reassure her. "We're just here to help. Everything you say is between you, me, and the doctor."

She blushed and nervously tucked her hair behind her ear.

"Ugh, I'm mortified. I have a heating pad on my chair at work because it's always freezing in my office. I've sat on it a million times and it's been fine, but today my butt started stinging like it was on fire."

"Uh oh," I said in anticipation.

"The heating pad burned a hole through my dress, and I think the skin on my butt is burned, too." Amber averted my gaze. "I made up some excuse and told my boss I had to work the rest of the day from home, then came directly here. I'm too scared to look at how bad it is."

"How long did you sit on the heating pad?" I asked.

"Not even ten minutes."

"And what setting was it on, low or high?"

"High, same as I always have it."

I placed a folded blue patient drape on the bed beside her. "Okay, I'm going to do an exam and come up with a treatment plan. If you'll take off everything from the waist down and just put the drape over your lap, I'll be back in a few minutes."

I stepped out and took a piece of printer paper from my white coat pocket. I scribbled some shorthand for my history of present illness (HPI): *CC burn on buttocks. Sat on heating pad for <10 min, high setting, stinging pain, burned through dress.*

When I opened the door to reenter Amber's room, I stopped dead in my tracks, mouth agape. The thick sea-green curtain that hung as a privacy screen in the room was now wrapped around Amber's waist three times over. She was standing in the middle of the room with it on like a toga. Apparently, she'd misunderstood my instructions to cover herself with the drape. I looked toward the bed. The paper drape I'd given her still lay folded and untouched.

Chief Complaint: "I cut my chin open"

I sutured my first laceration at 3:00 a.m. in the emergency department. A police officer accompanied an 18-year-old woman with a blood-soaked towel pressed to her chin. She was barefoot, and the lower half of her face was streaked with a mess of reds from lipstick and blood. The resident supervising me indicated for her to take a seat on the exam table, and she temporarily removed the towel from her chin to push herself up onto the cold, steel surface. Fresh blood smeared across the table.

I moved closer to examine the woman's wound: a large gash extended from the tip of her chin to the base of her throat. Before we suture the skin, we inject lidocaine or a similar anesthetic into the area to numb it. This is typically the most painful part of the repair; lidocaine burns, and most people scream or cuss when it goes in. Even the police officer averted his eyes briefly when I injected it. The young woman, Maria, barely flinched as the medicine entered her still-bleeding chin.

After I tested the skin with tweezers to ensure that it was numb, the resident nodded for me to get started. The most common way medical and PA students learned and practiced new medical skills was referred to as "see one, do one, teach one." We observed while an attending or resident performed a procedure, then performed it ourselves under supervision on the next appropriate occasion. This was how I performed my first lumbar puncture, paracentesis, splinting of a broken bone, and now, sutures. I had practiced on a plastic model once upon a time in Didactic Year, and that was it. I was slow and careful with the stitches and made conversation with Maria to distract attention from my awkward, inexperienced hands. She was nice and patient with me, but I could see how I wouldn't want to get on her bad side once she shared the details of her injury with me.

"I got into it with a girl at the ice-skating rink because she thought I was flirting with her boyfriend," she told me, rolling her eyes. "Girls always jump to conclusions because I'm hot. It's not a crime to talk to someone, even if he has a girlfriend. It's not like we were making out or humping each other."

"She came up to you and confronted you?" I asked. Maria's eyes flashed.

"Bitch shoved me from behind while I was skating. I fell and split my chin open on the ice."

I cringed. "Sorry. That had to hurt so badly."

Maria smirked and swung her legs against the exam table.

"You should see the other girl. She and her friends were all laughing until her boyfriend came over to see if I was okay. She almost lost her shit when he carried me off the ice. Then I grabbed my stiletto and hit her right in the middle of her forehead, like this."

I pulled my needle driver back just as Maria swung her arm inches from my face like she was throwing a 120-mile-per-hour pitch at a baseball game. The resident and the police officer both cried out in protest.

"Relax," Maria said, rolling her eyes again and waving them away. "You took my shoes away already, remember? Anyway," she said, turning her attention back to me, "I got her again on the cheek. There was blood everywhere. She accused me of assault, so they took my stiletto because it was the 'weapon.' She's probably getting more stitches than me right now."

Maria proudly concluded her victory speech, the moral of which was that a lot of women needed to just get over themselves and not get bent out of shape when a woman hotter than them talked to their boyfriends. My resident inspected my first-time handiwork on her chin and, satisfied, handed Maria back to the police officer. Once she got her stilettos back, it probably wouldn't be long before she was on her way to the other girl's house to finish the fight.

Chief Complaint: *Foreign body, pediatric*

In medicine, a foreign body is any object that's lodged somewhere it's not supposed to be. It could be a piece of glass stuck in someone's foot, a popcorn kernel stuck in a child's ear, or a piece of gauze left in a patient's body during surgery. It's a fairly common chief complaint in the ED.

One afternoon, a father brought his 6-year-old son in. The little one appeared quite comfortable—"in no acute distress", in medical lingo—and looked up from the video he was watching on an iPad when I entered the room.

"So, what's going on today, Chase?" I asked him.

"I swallowed a quarter," he replied, practically beaming as he patted his belly.

"You swallowed a quarter! How did that happen?"

"It's kind of my fault," the father interjected hastily. "I was bragging about how my frat brothers and I used to do stupid dares. I swallowed a bunch of coins because, you know, it just seems like a good idea when you're twenty and you've been drinking all day. I didn't think he'd actually do it."

So that's what actually goes on in frat houses. At least Chase was only six, not twenty.

I listened, amused, as the father related how he left the room that morning to grab an umbrella after he told Chase about his glory days. He didn't witness Chase's ingestion of the quarter firsthand.

"I dropped him off at school and he was acting normal," he

continued. "He didn't tell me he ate it until I picked him up this afternoon. Said he got it from his piggy bank."

I listened to Chase's actively gurgling belly with my stethoscope and palpated to make sure it was nontender. His vital signs were normal, and he had had no nausea, abdominal pain, or bowel movements since he swallowed the quarter earlier. Even though he looked comfortable and happy as a clam, I ordered an x-ray for good measure. You can never be too careful with kids; they can appear healthy one minute and rapidly deteriorate the next.

"I see it, Daddy!" Chase's eyes lit up as I pointed to the round, white shape on the x-ray and he looked to his father for approval. There was the quarter in all its glory. It was hard to hide the smile that crept up at the corners of my mouth.

I reassured Chase's father that the x-ray showed no signs of obstruction or perforation, and that Chase would likely poop out the quarter within the next couple of days. His father was relieved as he still hadn't told Chase's mother yet about what happened. He thanked me, sternly told Chase not to ingest any more money, and they went on their way.

Chief Complaint: Foreign body, adult

One Friday night, a 47-year-old man named Mr. Maldonado showed up for, according to his chart, a "rectal FB." According to him, he just had rectal pain and severe constipation, but once I informed him that the first step was a digital rectal exam, he pleaded for a sedative and told me he'd gotten an object stuck up there while he and his girlfriend were having sex. What object, he wouldn't say, but they had tried everything for the past six hours and couldn't remove it. Could we just put him to sleep and flush it out?

I presented the history to my attending, Dr. Stechler, who listened with a condescending look on his face.

"How old is this guy? Forty-five?"

"Forty-seven," I corrected him politely.

"So, old enough to know we're going to eventually figure out what it is, and still trying to be secretive about it," he remarked.

Before I had a chance to answer, Dr. Stechler swept past me, his white coat sending a breeze across my cheek as I followed behind like a dog scampering after its owner. A sandwich that was supposed to be my lunch was still sitting in my own coat pocket, squished against a foldable clipboard and a copy of *Pocket Medicine*. I hadn't had a moment to sit down that afternoon, between the patient who came in with the skin on the left side of his body barely clinging to him after a motorcycle accident, the patient who was 33 weeks pregnant with vaginal bleeding, the patient with a COPD exacerbation who we thought had left AMA (against medical advice) but had simply wandered outside to smoke some cigarettes, an illegal immigrant who had a virulent case of chicken pox and several impatient police officers huddled outside his isolation room, and a patient who I had been interviewing for all of five minutes for a chief complaint of "cough" when a nurse burst into the room, handed me an N95 mask, and pushed the patient's gurney into another isolation room. (Apparently, this last patient was suspected of having active TB. I shuddered; he had been coughing and hacking audibly for several hours, separated from other patients only by curtains. He said it had been like this for the past month, and I figured he had pneumonia or lung cancer or something.)

As I watched Dr. Stechler stride towards Mr. Maldonado's room, I realized that I had never seen him eat. He was always on the move and seemed to subsist solely off Diet Coke and adrenaline. He explained to Mr. Maldonado in no uncertain terms that this was a busy emergency department where patients waited for hours, and we worked around the clock to solve their problems so that the fewest possible number died.

Foreign bodies in the rectum needed to be removed promptly to prevent perforation of the intestines and a complicated surgery, and this was not the time or place to be embarrassed and secretive.

In his too-small hospital gown and with a thin drape across his lap, Mr. Maldonado remained closemouthed, and all we got out of him was that it wasn't a vibrator, bottle, or an object containing metal (we would be able to see these on an x-ray; materials like wood and plastic are often not visible). Although neither Dr. Stechler nor I could see the foreign body on our exam, Dr. Stechler could feel it with the fingertip of his glove. An x-ray was unrevealing, although at least it confirmed a lack of perforation. Dr. Stechler announced that we were going to remove the object manually. No general anesthesia. We needed Mr. Maldonado to remain awake so that he could bear down, as if he were having a bowel movement, and encourage the object further along.

After I numbed the area up and placed the retractor to Dr. Stechler's satisfaction, he positioned himself next to me with forceps in hand. I felt like a witness to the world's first man going through labor; Mr. Maldonado had to lie on his back with his knees high to his chest, scrunching up his face and pushing until the veins in his forehead bulged. Dr. Stechler peered intently into Mr. Maldonado's rectum and then, after several minutes, carefully extracted a yellowish-brown, pulpy object. *I hope that's not a piece of poop*, I thought as Dr. Stechler dropped it into the specimen container I held ready. How could he tell that was a foreign body?

I needn't have been worried with such amateur questions. Dr. Stechler presently grasped the remainder of the object, removed it in one elegant motion, and deposited it on top of the other piece in the container. Our curiosity was finally sated: it was half of a cucumber. I stood over the procedure tray, staring wordlessly. *Were Mr. Maldonado and his girlfriend just like, 'this sex is mind-blowing—but wait, let's check the fridge'?*

Dr. Stechler's voice broke through my thoughts about how an unsuspecting vegetable had become a sex toy.

"Looks like we're finished here," he said with an amused smirk to what looked like a seriously emotionally-wounded version of Mr. Maldonado. Then Dr. Stechler turned to me with an air of seriousness. "Emily, send the order to pathology so they can get a good read on it."

Chief Complaint: Wound, left hand

One morning, an ED nurse told me that a 50-year-old man was here for a wound on his left hand. When I entered the room, the man was sitting miserably with a mountain of gauze about a foot thick wrapped around his hand. His arm looked more like a stick of cotton candy than a human extremity. He grimaced as I unwound the gauze and examined the bloody wound.

"How did this happen, Mr. Vernon?" I asked.

Mr. Vernon hesitated before relaying the day's events in a subdued and sheepish voice. At 2:00 a.m. he awoke to shouting and rustling outside his bedroom window. He took his gun out of his nightstand drawer and made his way around the entire perimeter of the house. But he didn't see anyone.

After crouching behind the bushes for a few minutes, Mr. Vernon made his way back inside and sat down in his recliner. He still felt that something wasn't quite right, so he kept his gun ready in his lap just in case the person tried to come back or break in. At some point, Mr. Vernon fell asleep.

At 5:00 a.m., his alarm went off for work. Startled, Mr. Vernon jumped awake. His finger was still on the trigger, the gun went off in his hand, and the bullet went through his left palm.

I took in Mr. Vernon's story with a calm, neutral expression on my face, even as my eyes felt like they were going to pop out of my head. The nurse had forgotten to mention that the most salient detail in his chief complaint wasn't just *wound* but *gunshot wound*. Fortunately, Mr. Vernon's vital signs were stable, and the accident happened more than an hour ago. He couldn't think of anyone who might have ill will toward him, and thought maybe what he'd heard had simply been a stray dog or cat.

Mr. Vernon seemed believable, but a part of me still wondered if someone else had shot him. I'd caught him glancing over his shoulder earlier, like he was still looking for the mysterious person who had been creeping around his house.

"No one else was involved?" I asked.

He shook his head.

"Did you call 911?"

Again, he shook his head no.

"I didn't want the cops to know. They probably wouldn't believe that I shot myself, and they might take my gun away. You don't have to turn me in, do you? I mean, since I didn't hurt anyone?" Mr. Vernon looked at me nervously, the pain in his hand temporarily forgotten. I'd lived in Texas long enough to know how much Texans love their Second Amendment rights.

"I don't need to 'turn you in' to anyone," I reassured him. So that was why he seemed uneasy. "This sounds like it was an accident, not a crime, and the only place it will say what happened is in your medical record. Bad news is, I think you're going to need surgery on your hand. I'm going to talk with the doctor, and we'll be back soon."

Mr. Vernon nodded rapidly, looking relieved.

"Yes, ma'am. I'll get whatever surgery you want me to have, just don't let them take away my guns."

Chief Complaint: "My wedding ring is stuck"

I had barely started my shift one evening when a young man burst through the main automatic doors. I glanced up from the patient notes I was reviewing and stuffed them in the pocket of my white coat.

"I need help!" the man shouted in the waiting area to no one in particular. Only the triage nurse sitting next to me seemed to notice him. She waved him over to the desk and whispered to me out the side of her mouth as he made his way over to us.

"He walked in by himself and he's not bleeding. Looks fine to me. Hello, sir. Driver's license, please. What brings you to the emergency department today?"

The man thrust the back of his hand into the nurse's face. He was breathing hard, his face red and sweaty.

"My wedding ring's stuck and it's cutting off my circulation," he huffed in a panic. Indeed, his left fourth finger was about three times the size of the others, and the swollen skin obscured part of the ring. The nurse shot him an annoyed look for invading her personal space and indicated for me to take him to a curtained-off area for evaluation once she entered his information.

"Can you tell me what happened, Mr. McClary?" I asked after we'd introduced ourselves.

"I caught my wife cheating and went to throw the ring at her. But it wouldn't come off and got stuck."

"How long has it been swollen like this?"

"I don't know, an hour maybe." Mr. McClary squirmed uncomfortably as I examined his hand. The skin was purplish-red, warm, tender, and he could not bend his finger. His wedding ring had effectively become a tourniquet.

"Has this ever happened before?" I continued, as we were taught to always ask. He looked at me like I had a third eye growing out of my forehead, but answered, nonetheless.

"No. I never take it off. The more I pulled, the more it swelled up . . . you can get it off, right?"

I met Mr. McClary's pleading eyes sympathetically and explained that the attending and I would do everything we could. *Could a ring be tight enough to amputate a person's finger?* I didn't know and tried not to think about it. All I knew was that his finger looked really bad. My attending repeated a quick physical exam and, after the shortest procedure consent I've ever been a part of ("Yes, cut it off, burn it off, do whatever you have to do, that woman is dead to me"), we got to work.

An hour went by as the attending and I tried unsuccessfully to remove the ring with a ring cutter (most EDs have one) and a pair of pliers I obtained from a hospital maintenance worker. I was growing increasingly apprehensive because the ring had not budged at all, while my attending was simply frustrated that Mr. McClary was still in his patient queue. We still had almost fifteen patients requiring our attention, and he'd estimated that this would only take half an hour at most. Of the three of us, at least Mr. McClary was calm now that his finger was numb from lidocaine and epinephrine. He seemed like a nice guy and we talked about his son, who played football in high school and who he was clearly super proud of.

Beads of sweat formed along the attending's hairline as he tried a third time with the pliers. No luck. His own hand was starting to look red from the effort.

"Do you know if your ring is made of titanium?" he asked Mr. McClary wearily.

"Yeah, I think that's what it's made of." Mr. McClary's face reddened again as his attention returned to the events that led him here. "My wife wanted something indestructible. She probably chose this on purpose."

The attending grunted and raised his eyebrows.

"Titanium is notoriously hard to cut," he explained to

both Mr. McClary and me. "If we can't do it with these, we may have to get you to another hospital."

"How do you cut titanium?" Mr. McClary asked, now exasperated.

"You need diamond-coated discs or tempered tool steel blades."

"You're speaking another language, doctor."

Agreed, I thought. *Definitely didn't learn about this in school.*

After another half hour of lubrication, ice, elevating Mr. McClary's hand, and a tourniquet, the ring finally slid off his finger, intact. As I felt the heavens open with hallelujahs, the attending indicated the ring and asked Mr. McClary, "Should I . . . get rid of this for you?" Mr. McClary scoffed.

"Nah. The second I get out of here, I'm going straight home and telling her we're getting a divorce. Then I'm going to fling this ring in her face."

Chief Complaint: GI Bleed and Unconscious

At 6:30 one morning, my attending physician stopped speaking to the medical student and me mid-sentence as the main ED doors flew open. A muscular man in scrubs knelt next to an elderly man on a moving gurney, performing CPR on him as paramedics wheeled them toward us. The paramedic in the lead shouted to my attending that the man was approximately eighty years old, unconscious, and had a massive gastrointestinal (GI) bleed. As we sprinted alongside the gurney, clearing a path through the packed corridor, the paramedic continued to describe the interventions his team had attempted so that ours could pick up right where they left off.

We entered a huge, dark room that resembled a warehouse. The slate-gray walls were bare except for a black rectangular clock near the ceiling that displayed the time in large red numbers. An operating table with an attached IV pole stood in the center of the room, while a large cabinet rested against one wall. As the paramedics handed the man off to the ED staff, a trauma nurse hissed for the medical student and me to make ourselves invisible and to stay out of the way.

It was as if we were on the sidelines of a war. The man in scrubs, a resident according to his ID badge, continued to perform CPR without pausing as staff transferred the unconscious patient from the gurney to the table. I'd practiced chest compressions on dummies before and found it relatively easy. The resident's muscles had muscles, and he looked exhausted. Sweat poured down his face and he exhaled forcefully as he maintained the compression rhythm. I suddenly felt unsure if I'd be able to do CPR on a real human if the need ever arose.

The patient briefly regained pulses, and I looked hopefully at the digital ticker tape overhead that showed ventricular tachycardia before the patient suddenly coded again. What seemed like twenty different people swarmed about, their bodies filling every inch of space around him, and orders rang through the air one after another. My attending placed a central line near the patient's collarbone while a resident inserted a separate line through the patient's groin. The resident who had been doing CPR finally took a break since others were now using a device to shock the man's heart. Other people hung bags of IV fluids on the pole and placed a tube down the patient's throat. Someone was shouting the blood type and quantity for a blood transfusion, and someone was shouting back. It was a blur of terrifying chaos, even though the medical team clearly knew the protocol and communicated effectively with one another.

Then, as quickly as the war started, it was over. Someone pronounced the time of death, and people stepped away from the table, sweating and breathing like they had just run a 5k. The clock showed that twenty-five minutes had passed since we first entered the room, but it seemed much shorter than that. The man had no identification on him, and a nurse was assigned to figure out who he was so they could notify family or next of kin.

Everyone seemed to leave the room at once. The trauma nurse who had addressed us earlier ushered the medical student and me out and said, "That's it. He's gone." I took one last look at the lifeless, nameless old man on the table before the doors closed behind us. I didn't feel repulsed, as I had by the cadavers in Gross Anatomy lab. The patient was still but there was no blood splattered anywhere. Tubes hung limply from several places on his body. He just looked like he was resting and might wake up any second.

My attending had already moved on and stood talking to another patient. He jerked his head slightly for me to join him and the medical student at the bedside. I swallowed hard, my mouth dry like I had inhaled dust. I didn't know what to feel, to think. It was the first time I'd seen someone die, the first time I'd seen someone perform CPR on a living person and not a dummy in a CPR certification class. *Who was he? What were they going to do with his body? Shouldn't we at least observe a moment of silence or something?* The man's last seconds of life, while certainly traumatic, were also an all-consuming, orchestrated effort fueled by the medical team's heart for a complete stranger. He was surrounded by people who cared even though he didn't know them. I didn't know whether I should be thankful or sad about that.

In a daze, I made my way over to the new patient, introduced myself, and caught up on the details of his story. We smiled and emanated warmth to show that we were fully invested, and never once stopped or spoke about what we had just witnessed. There were always more living people who needed our help.

CLINICAL YEAR: SURGERY

The American College of Surgeons recognizes fourteen surgical specialties, two of which I encountered during clinical year: general surgery and neurosurgery. While all physicians must tread carefully in matters of life and death, surgeons bear additional weight on their shoulders. It isn't enough to have manual dexterity and an expert understanding of human anatomy. Normal human variation, underlying disease, and chance contribute just as much to whether a patient has a successful outcome after surgery. A neurosurgeon's inadvertent mistake could be the difference between improved function and paralysis. But even if a neurosurgeon makes no mistakes, a patient who wakes up coherent after brain surgery may unexpectedly suffer a stroke or die days later. The fact that surgeons accept this and still perform surgery made them an entirely different breed of physicians in my mind.

I arrived at the Houston VA Hospital's expansive parking lot every day at 4:00 a.m. for my general surgery rotation. The first surgery of the day was always between 5:00 a.m. and 6:00 a.m., and we reviewed our patients' current statuses and treatment plans beforehand, which is called rounding. There were cholecystectomies (gallbladder removals), hernia repairs, a surgery to drain an abscess after a man swallowed a tiny fishbone and it perforated his liver … oh, and more cholecystectomies. Even ten years later, cholecystectomies remain in the top three outpatient surgeries performed in the United States.

I had barely started rounds one morning when the second-year resident called me aside.

"Hi, Jeff," I greeted him.

"Hey. Get two coffees downstairs for us at Starbucks." *Us* meaning him and the chief resident, who had both worked for thirty hours straight without sleeping and still had twelve more hours on the clock.

Resident interactions with students were always that way. Unsmiling orders, no pleases or thank-yous, no additional details. They often tasked us with "scutwork," activities that had nothing to do with learning medicine. *Why can't you get your own coffee? Do I have to use my own money for it? Where should I find you afterward?* I often felt like I was working under the megalomaniacal fashion editor-in-chief Miranda Priestly from *The Devil Wears Prada*: "Please, bore someone else with your ... questions." I'm pretty sure Jeff still didn't know my name, even though we had spent twelve hours a day together for the last two weeks. There was no point for surgery residents to learn the names of their little minions; students came and went every four weeks, while residents endured unceasing work and brutal hours with no respite for five years.

As brusque as the younger residents were, however, the general surgery chief resident, Ewan, put them all to shame. Ewan knew only one mode and volume of communication (shouting), cursed like a sailor, and fired questions at us like he did not have time for our answers. I felt like I had unwittingly joined the ROTC. He was 1,000 percent unapologetic and no-nonsense. The rest of my team described him with a variety of less polite names: condescending asshole, prick, inhuman monster, motherfucker with a superiority complex.

I marveled at the cutthroat perfectionism and technical skill that Ewan must possess to become a surgical chief resident. A parade of surgeries from 5:00 a.m. to 4:00 p.m.

Monday through Saturday demanded his undivided attention, precision, and stamina. Most days, he did not see the sun; the operating rooms were dark and windowless. He rarely saw his wife or his two young boys and survived solely on coffee and bottles of 5-hour Energy. Most nights, he was lucky if he slept for three consecutive hours because he was on call. He stayed in the resident on-call room of the hospital, a bare, depressing room with two twin-sized beds. Ewan clearly strove to be the best, come hell or high water, which meant the most surgeries under his belt and the fewest deaths, and surgery before everything else in his life. The ungodly hours and workload would never permit a life outside of the hospital anyway. It was quite the opposite of the work-life balance I imagined for myself. I saw Ewan as overworked, under pressure, sleep-deprived … but still human.

On one occasion, after the anesthesiologist sedated a patient for surgery, Ewan instructed me to insert a Foley catheter into the man's penis. Patients cannot control urination when they are under general anesthesia, so the catheter empties the bladder during surgery and prevents a mess. I had never inserted a catheter before and told him as much.

"You don't need anyone to show you," Ewan said, waving aside the preposterous suggestion. "You just choke the chicken and shove it in. It's like a hand job."

"Right." *I don't know what kind of hand jobs you're used to.* I put a pair of gloves on and pulled back the bedsheet so it rested on the unconscious patient's knees.

"Good god, you don't need gloves for that," Ewan snapped impatiently. He reached in front of me and unceremoniously tossed up the patient's hospital gown, which exposed a small, shriveled, uncircumcised penis that looked like a gray turd. *Yep, I'm keeping the gloves on.* I pushed the foreskin back with my left hand and inserted the rubber tubing into the opening at the end of what felt like a semi-solid piece of diarrhea. The catheter went in easily for the first several inches, but then I felt the flaccid penis slither from my grasp as if intentionally trying to evade the unwanted intrusion. I remembered the warnings I had learned about injuring the urethra or causing bleeding and started to loosen my grip to reposition my left hand.

Ewan suddenly grabbed my wrist, commanding me to tighten my grip instead and hold the foreskin back with more force.

"Damn it, just shove it in!" he thundered. "You're not going to hurt him—he's unconscious."

I followed orders and finished the job, thinking how it would have been a hell of a lot easier to insert a long-ass tube into a man's penis if it weren't a limp noodle. Still, I thanked Ewan for letting me do my first catheterization because that's the kind of glamorous stuff you've got to do to become a PA.

During the surgery rotation, we also routinely assisted in the operating room (OR) by holding retractors, metal instruments that keep the body cavity open so that the surgeon has a clear view and space to work. We maneuvered the retractors around vital organs and blood vessels at the surgeon's command, sometimes standing in the same spot for several hours as our arms ached and tingled to maintain the necessary resistance. No point in exerting mental energy on this, though; we had to remind ourselves constantly of the rules of the OR, like not locking our knees while standing and not obstructing anyone's path to or view of the operating area. Most importantly, we were hyper-focused on sterile procedure, a violation of which was practically punishable by death. When part of the patient's body is open during surgery, any germ from the environment can cause infection and lead to potential disability or death. To avoid exposing the patient, sterile procedure is expected of anyone, participant or observer, who enters an OR suite.

The protocols began as soon as we entered the OR antechamber. Scrubbing-in was a religious process of covering the head, face, and nearly the entire body with clean gear. After scrubbing our arms and hands in a specified pattern for a specified amount of time, we held them in front of us and away from the body, letting the water drip onto the floor as we entered the OR so it wouldn't touch our scrubs. The scrub nurses provided us with the materials to dry, gown, and glove ourselves, each subsequent layer more constricting. By necessity, scrub nurses kept a tight ship because they were primarily responsible for enforcing sterile procedure from start to finish. One wrong move (scrubbing our hands for too short or too long, drying an area of skin we'd already dried with the towel, turning our back on the sterile operating field), and they unleashed the Wrath of God. Whether it was one minute or 120 minutes into the surgery, a break in sterile procedure meant a possible infection for the patient and an automatic exit from the OR for the perpetrator back into the antechamber to restart the scrubbing-in process. My first week, I was sent back once, fortunately before the surgery commenced, and learned not to overthink the process. One poor student got sent out three times before he got the hang of it, partly because he got more nervous each time about not messing up.

During a routine hernia repair, Ewan selected me to assist. The only problem: I could barely see over the top of the operating table, being only 5'2", and he had the table at elbow height, which for him was about 5'0". When I had asked the OR scrub nurse earlier for something to stand on, she had glared at me like she wanted the last five seconds of her life back and denied my request. I'd grown accustomed to these kinds of responses during the rotation, so I resigned myself to my current predicament. To the scrub nurses, we were clumsy idiots who fumbled their way through scrubbing-in protocols, always got in the way, and asked inane questions or else took forever suturing up the patient's incision site after surgery (this increases the duration of both the surgery and general anesthesia, which is associated with its own risks). I tried to be empathetic. While we students would move on to another setting in four weeks, the scrub nurses weathered the chief resident's yelling on a year-round basis and didn't have the reserves to deal with our special requests.

Ewan presently reached over to hand me a retractor and instead almost whacked me in the face.

"Why the hell are you down there?" he bellowed. "Someone get this girl a fucking stepstool!"

"We don't have stepstools in this OR because no one's that fucking short." The scrub nurse spat out each word like it was poison, and laser beams shot from her eyes as she stared me down for inconveniencing everyone with my height. Still, she knew better than to disobey Ewan.

The minutes ticked by painfully until she eventually secured a stepstool and threw it at my feet, her experienced aim causing it to be just inches from breaking the sterile field. I held my arms up in front of my body as I climbed onto it, to avoid contaminating myself or the active operating area, and maneuvered sideways so that I wouldn't have my back to the field at any time.

Ewan was silent and noticeably sullen for the remainder of the operation. He handed the task of closing up the patient to the resident instead of to me as he'd done in the past.

I thanked the scrub nurse when I exited but instead was met with another icy glare.

"Get out; I need to clean up," she growled.

My neurosurgery rotation wasn't quite as emotionally charged. My attending, Dr. Lombardi, had operated for more than thirty years in private practice and was poised and content at this juncture in life. His residency days in the distant past, he enjoyed the hours, clientele, and posh lifestyle his work afforded him. His practiced technique was second nature, like he could have performed it just as expertly in his sleep. However, Dr. Lombardi confessed that each surgery was still an intimidating beast, with stakes so high it could break his being if he dwelled on them. It was with this complex mix of humility, fear, and determination—which themselves arise exclusively from the brain—that he entered each of his patients' brains. Somehow, Dr. Lombardi always found a way to slide a joke or sly remark in as he did this serious work. His sense of humor sharply contrasted with the rage that defined the general surgery chief resident, who was always just one procedure away from blowing his stack.

One afternoon, Dr. Lombardi performed a brain aneurysm repair for a man in his fifties. This was the last patient on the schedule that day, and everyone was in good spirits because we had stayed relatively on time. I was legitimately shocked when the scrub nurse asked me about my weekend plans; this kind of banal chitchat was unheard of in the VA general surgery unit.

About halfway through the procedure, Dr. Lombardi suddenly set his instruments down and walked wordlessly over to the glass window separating the OR from the antechamber. He said something in a serious tone over the microphone to the woman on the other side. My non-surgeon eyes hadn't noticed any obvious complications, and no one else in the room appeared concerned. At least, no alarms were going off, and no blood was spilling onto the floor. I looked at the anesthesiologist: he was engrossed in a book and had his surgical booties propped up on his desk.

Suddenly, the music that had been playing loudly in the OR stopped. In the following silence, I heard a series of clicks over the speakers that sounded like a shuffle of an old-school iPod. Dr. Lombardi, who had since gone to the antechamber and scrubbed in again, returned to his position at the operating table as a new song burst forth. It sounded familiar . . . . Dr. Lombardi picked up his instruments and got right back to work as if nothing happened.

"The music is critical," he said after a few moments, as if imparting the secret to performing surgery successfully. "That last song just didn't feel right."

"Okay," I said. He held up an instrument and I fell silent. "Here comes the chorus. It's the best part."

I listened as Leona Lewis belted out:

> *You cut me open and I*
> *Keep bleeding, keep, keep bleeding love*
> *I keep bleeding, I keep, keep bleeding love*
> *Keep bleeding, keep, keep bleeding love...*

The regionally renowned neurosurgeon looked up as if gauging the team's level of approval at his song choice.

"Just need to make sure the patient doesn't keep bleeding," he quipped with his signature laugh.

Another morning, I watched as the anesthesiologist sedated a 40-year-old woman for a spine procedure. After she drifted off to la la land, the team strapped her to a backboard and, in one smooth motion, flipped her over onto her stomach and onto the operating table. They covered her upper body with drapes, leaving only a square of exposed skin on her neck for the sterile operating field. A tattoo of two intertwined female gender symbols stared up at us. The first incision had to go right between the two symbols, and Dr. Lombardi raised an eyebrow at me over the top of his mask.

"Wonder what this lady would do if we sewed her neck

back up and the tattoo was just slightly off so they're not holding hands anymore," he said deviously. I cringed, unsure of the appropriate response.

"I'm just kidding," he said with a laugh as he lowered his scalpel to her skin. "You don't do that unless you want to get sued. I knew that woman who was with her looked butch though!"

After some time, Dr. Lombardi spoke more seriously of what other patients' tattoos had taught him.

"Years ago, this guy came through the ER with the bottom half of his arm all mangled after a motorcycle accident. We took him to surgery to see if we could save the nerve. The anesthesiologist pulled up the patient's sleeve, and there's a swastika covering his entire tricep. It was, you know, disturbing." I looked up at him, wide-eyed, but Dr. Lombardi's eyes and hands were steady and focused on the patient. With practiced ease, he readjusted one of the retractors as he recalled the uproar the discovery caused.

"Some of my nurses said I shouldn't do the surgery at all, and several of them left the room once I decided to do it. I didn't have a choice. We're not going to have the same religious or political or even humanitarian views as our patients, but we always have a duty to them."

"Wow, that's tough," I remarked. "I don't know what I would have done."

"I think you would have done the same thing," Dr. Lombardi replied matter-of-factly, as if he was familiar with my character after only knowing me for two weeks. "We didn't go into medicine to only help certain people."

"I guess that's true," I conceded.

Although I was twenty-three years old, I couldn't help but feel like a child as I listened to the wise words this benevolent, grandfatherly man imparted. I certainly knew more medical information and skills than when I started PA school, but I still understood so little about the human condition and the ethical challenges of my profession. This right here, it occurred to me, was the very reason for medical hierarchies and pimping and all the other things that my peers and I often griped about as unfair and demeaning. PA and medical students went into clinical rotations with the same amount of experience, which was none, and trained together in preparation for how, one day, we would also work together in clinics and hospitals. As naïve as we were, we somehow also felt confidently entitled to respect, recognition, and instruction. We received ample but essential doses of humility. We became accustomed to a constant state of discomfort, of sink or swim, and, even more often than *see one, do one, teach one*, of *see zero and just do one*. Clinical rotations were the great equalizer, and offered the first, small glimpses into our futures as clinicians.

PART II
THE EARLY YEARS

GREEN IN A WHITE COAT

December 1 was Graduation Day, and a muggy 90 degrees in Houston. As I fidgeted with my cap and tried to remember which side the tassel went on, I was a mess of emotions: eager to join the ranks of the professors who would present me with my diploma, hopeful about all the future patients I would help, excited to move to Dallas for my first job at an urgent care clinic. At the same time, low-grade dread hummed beneath the surface. Graduation Day meant that the five-hour Physician Assistant National Certifying Exam (PANCE) was officially only two weeks away. It felt like cruel irony to overshadow such a momentous day with the most challenging obstacle still ahead. I would have to curtail celebrations with loved ones and become a recluse fueled by caffeine, grit, and practice questions.

The brief interlude between graduation and boards wasn't a coincidence. Studying and test-taking would still be second nature. For what was the greatest survival skill the Baylor PA curriculum had taught us, if not the ability and stamina to take multiple choice exams (eight exams every eight weeks during Didactic Year!) until we went cross-eyed?

"Baylor's PA students perform; we've prepared them," the program director had declared proudly a few weeks back as handouts had gone around the classroom. We silently processed the table comparing the most recent graduating classes' first-time pass rates for the PANCE:

100%
100%
98%
100%

"They don't think we're stressed out enough?" one of my classmates, Lance, muttered beside me as the director started digging for something behind the podium.

Allison, another classmate, quickly did the math in her head and somberly told us, "If that class had forty people like ours did, 98% means only one person failed that year."

"Baylor probably banned that person from alumni reunions," Lance responded sarcastically. He addressed our row in a louder voice: "Guys, let me just apologize now if I'm the one who brings our average down. You can put my mugshot next to our class's score."

I laughed along, but a heaviness arose in the pit of my stomach that would live there for the next several weeks. I was at least slightly afraid of being that one person. The PANCE was 300 questions, and we had one minute to complete each question. While my classmates were all Speedy Gonzaleses on tests, I routinely consumed the last thirty minutes before time was up painstakingly going over every answer I had marked "unsure." I was especially susceptible to phrases like *which one of the following DOES NOT ...* or *which of the following is NOT true?* Inexplicably, they would put the language center of my brain on pause so that I could not simultaneously reconcile scientific knowledge. I compensated by compulsively reading and rereading the questions, which was as time-consuming as it was tedious.

The weeks following graduation were a blur. Chug coffee, study, block out the noise, try to rest even though images and practice questions floated before my eyelids when I closed them at night. On PANCE day, dutifully wear the test center's noise-canceling headphones so I wouldn't be distracted or discouraged by the sounds of chairs emptying around me. We had the option to take a break between each block of sixty questions, but some classmates went straight through and finished before I had even started the final block. Afterwards, we packed up our apartments like weary soldiers moving camp. Most of my classmates would return to their home states. I said my goodbyes, and headed, sleep-deprived, up US-75 to my new home in Dallas.

At the end of December and two PANCE website crashes later, I would finally see that single, glorious word on my computer screen: *passed*. The elation that overcame me would remain unsurpassed for another four years, when my now-husband would ask me to marry him. I swapped out my short white coat for the long one reserved for PAs and physicians, proudly admiring the new credentials of PA-C embroidered behind my name: Physician Assistant–Certified. My newly-purchased business professional clothes hung beside it in the closet, cheerfully in denial about the $45,000 of grad school loans I'd racked up by this point.

And then I was flying solo. I saw my first patient, then my first ten and my first fifty. I was thrilled when I knew diagnoses and treatments without needing to consult any references. Other times, I felt like a skilled impostor who spoke and moved with assuredness in the exam room before covertly seeking the counsel of my supervising physician on the other side of the door. Dr. Dorsanio was my lifeline. Pensive, decisive, and always dressed as if he had just stepped out of *GQ Magazine*, he was generous with his time and expertise. He was also the only one who knew that a multiple-choice exam and a couple of months were all that separated Emily the Student from Emily the Healthcare Professional. He emphasized that although I may still be green, I couldn't let patients suspect that. Even when I felt the opposite, I would put on a façade of confidence, keep up with the current medical evidence, and learn from my mistakes so as not to repeat them. I wore the white coat now; with that came expectations of knowledge, experience, and certainty.

Drew Agostini
23yo M
Chief Complaint: "I bit my tongue really hard"

    One morning, a young man named Drew came in with a tongue laceration. I couldn't see the injury at first because his mouth was full of blood. With Dr. Dorsanio's assistance, I applied pressure to his tongue to reduce the bleeding and get a proper look: the front third was nearly separated from the back portion.
    In excruciating and halting statements, Drew explained that he accidentally bit his tongue while doing push-ups in his apartment. He immediately collapsed on the ground from pain and hit his chin, and his teeth cut deeper through the thickest part of his tongue. When Drew called his roommate, the latter couldn't understand him over the phone due to his new and severe lisp. Panicked and about to pass out from the blinding pain, Drew couldn't think of any other solution but to drive himself the thirty minutes to our urgent care clinic. He texted his roommate, who also raced here, and both were absolutely terrified that Drew's tongue was unsalvageable.
    I tried to sound reassuring as I promised Drew that we would help put his tongue back together. By we, I meant the closest emergency department after I consulted its ear, nose, and throat (ENT) service, because "refer to ENT" was the textbook answer for this scenario. Surely, surgery that could

impair speech, swallowing, or appearance should be left to a specialist, and not to a PA with only a handful of non-tongue laceration repairs under her belt.

Dr. Dorsanio listened quietly to my treatment plan outside the room, then informed me that we would be taking care of anything short of a tongue that was completely cut off and outside of the patient's mouth. This wasn't the answer I was expecting. My own mouth felt dry with nervous anticipation as we discussed the procedure, including anesthesia technique and suture choice. The *see one, do one, teach one* days of clinicals apparently weren't over.

"I'll stand by for the anesthesia. Any other questions and you know I'll be there right away," Dr. Dorsanio told me seriously.

I nodded and took a deep breath. I had thought that this was a one-way PA-supervising physician relationship, in which I trusted him to know everything and became his mentee. It dawned on me that Dr. Dorsanio also trusted me to recognize when his intervention or assistance was necessary, before a complication arose. Indeed, he had been true to his word since we started working together. Even in those instances when my concerns were trivial or easily resolved, he had always stopped what he was doing and made himself available to me.

We re-entered the room, and I doubt Drew heard much of what I said as I obtained his consent for the procedure. He merely nodded and whimpered, trying to fight back the tears that streamed down his cheeks. He probably thought whatever came next could not possibly hurt as much as lacerating his tongue. Even without the tormented scream that issued from his chest when I injected lidocaine into the back of his mouth, the agony in his eyes and the thrashing of his legs made me feel like I had betrayed him. I gritted my teeth, keeping a firm grip on the syringe.

"It's almost over, man," the roommate choked out, keeping a steady hand on Drew's arm even as he turned his head away and squeezed his eyes shut. He deserved a medal for friendship and for trying to convince Drew that it was almost over when it hadn't even started. Although Drew and I were about the same age, I involuntarily soothed him as I would a child. I told him what a good job he was doing and that it wouldn't hurt much longer. Dr. Dorsanio looked vaguely amused by our interactions; he had undoubtedly seen much worse trauma in his years as an urgent care physician. My coddling marked a sharp contrast between the veteran doctor and the amateur PA.

Mercifully, the anesthetic kicked in a few minutes later. Dr. Dorsanio left us, again reiterating to me, "Come get me if you need anything." I nodded and reached for the instruments on the procedure tray.

Once Drew relaxed a bit, his roommate told me a story about a different occasion when Drew showcased his pushups without hurting himself.

"He put on his resume under 'skills' that he could do a hundred and fifty pushups, and they asked to see it at a job interview. He's an engineer, by the way. Drew's like, 'You want me to do it in my suit and tie?' and they told him, 'You can take your coat off first.' So he takes his coat off and just drops and gives them a hundred and fifty, no sweat." The roommate glanced at me, apparently to gauge my level of awe.

"Wow," I remarked, minimally impressed but going along with it to keep Drew distracted. "Did he get the job?"

"No, he didn't get that one. But the interviewer did give him props for doing what he said he could do. He was going to stop him after twenty pushups, but then just let it happen because no one had ever done pushups at an interview before."

Bros, I thought as I smiled wryly. *I would never dream of including pushups on my resume. Not that I could do even twenty pushups if I tried, but come on, that's not what they mean by "skills."*

The repair went smoothly, and I was grateful Dr. Dorsanio

had discussed the specifics with me beforehand. Even though I had never done this particular procedure, our brief conversation and anatomy review provided a certain degree of confidence. I knew how to administer local anesthesia already; this was just a new location. I knew how to suture, too; the texture of this surface just felt very different from those that overlay bony body parts. Dr. Dorsanio had not recklessly handed me the reins. He had challenged me to think like a professional, to accept that I would encounter many more unfamiliar clinical situations that were nevertheless within my "scope of practice."

After I finished suturing, the sterile drape around Drew's mouth was so bloody that he looked like a victim in a gory horror movie. I was pleased with the finished product, though, and fetched Dr. Dorsanio, who subtly indicated his approval and removed the drape from Drew's face. To my surprise, he had fallen asleep underneath it. Drew's roommate and I looked at each other, and I debated for a moment whether to wake Drew up since he was clearly exhausted after the day's traumatic events. The man just wanted to do some pushups.

Confidential
29yo M
Chief Complaint: Left eye pain

Under Dr. Dorsanio's tutelage, I also learned the various nuances of patient confidentiality. We were legally required to keep at least eighteen distinct pieces of protected health information (PHI) private. This included not only a patient's name and birthdate, but also photos, phone numbers, email addresses, and dates of hospital admissions—anything that could potentially identify someone. Hundreds of patients passed through our clinic every day, so we were responsible for preventing them from seeing or overhearing other patients' information. Early on, Dr. Dorsanio cautioned me to always confirm who, if anyone, a patient had authorized us to share health information with. For instance, if a woman asked me what I had prescribed for her husband or what his test results were, I had better be 100 percent sure her name was on her husband's authorization form. It didn't matter if they were legally married. If the husband had written only his brother's name on the form, I couldn't utter a single word about his care to his wife.

Even if a patient was a celebrity and we were dying to tell everyone we knew, confidentiality was paramount. I still remember the morning a nurse named Dana led a patient to one of the exam rooms. The other nurses, who had previously been in an animated conversation in the hallway, suddenly fell silent. I glanced up to see an impressively tall man, at least 6'5" by my estimations, duck slightly under a doorframe. I saw only the back of his head before he disappeared from view. Looked like a regular guy to me.

After a few minutes, Dana walked past me to her desk, fanning herself with a patient clipboard.

"Ooh Emily, he is *fine*! His wife is a lucky woman."

"Oh, Dana," I responded with a laugh. So that was why everyone had done a double take. Dana changed the patient's status in the system to "ready for provider" and briefly presented to me: "Chief complaint: foreign body in left eye since 9 a.m., thinks a little piece of metal got in it. Normal vision, but he has redness, swelling, and watering. Pain level 6 out of 10." She paused and added, "But he still looks like a 10 out of 10."

"I'll be sure to tell him you said that," I teased her, wiggling my eyebrows.

"You better make up a reason for me to come back in the room and assist with the exam," she fired back.

Upon entering the room, though, I promptly forgot our conversation. At first glance, the patient looked like someone had punched him in the face. His eye was nearly swollen shut, and he blotted it frequently with a bunched-up tissue. I introduced myself to him and his wife and reviewed their suspicions that a piece of metal had entered his eye. Neither had witnessed the injury.

I then turned off the lights and inspected both of the patient's eyes with an ophthalmoscope (first rule of physical examination: always examine the unaffected side first, then compare).

"Ughhh," the patient moaned, blinking excessively as he struggled to keep his left eye open. I stepped back and gave him a break from the bright light while his wife patted his hand sympathetically.

"I'm going to put some drops in to numb your eye, and then add dye to see if I can find the metal. Does that sound okay to you?" I asked.

"Whatever you need to do. I just want it to stop hurting," the patient answered miserably.

"The drops should numb the pain for at least ten minutes," I said. "What do you do for work?" Several of my patients were welders; perhaps the stray piece of metal was from working with some type of machinery. The man, who up until this point had looked immensely pained and unhappy, turned to his wife and burst out laughing before he answered.

"I play basketball."

In the end, there was no metal. In fact, the dye revealed a corneal abrasion that I determined his contact lenses had caused. He occasionally forgot to take them out before he went to sleep, and this had been the case two nights ago. I provided prescriptions for both ciprofloxacin and diclofenac eye drops, and the patient and his wife thanked me profusely. As we emerged from the room, multiple employees who were "nonchalantly" hanging around to catch a glimpse of the patient suddenly tried to look busy. Dr. Dorsanio had reminded them that they were not to take photos, read the patient's chart, address him by name, or otherwise identify him without his permission because it would violate PHI. We must have looked like an odd pair, him at a towering 6'10" and me at a measly 5'2". It was probably for the best that I didn't know who he was, or I might not have been so cool and collected during his appointment.

So unfolded the days of my fledgling career. From fine-tuning my knowledge of disease processes to maintaining the confidentiality of pro basketball players, I was constantly learning, adjusting, evolving. Much of my growth happened behind the scenes, and I credit Dr. Dorsanio for his exacting and compassionate mentorship. He took on the daunting task of smoothing out my rough edges in both the practice and the art of medicine, and nurtured the critical thinking and clinical judgment that was starting to develop. Without his guidance, I would not have become the practitioner I am today.

LEARNING FROM THE BEST

As the months went by, I worked with several other physicians. Since our urgent care clinic only accepted walk-ins, bottlenecks resulted when patients came in more quickly than clinicians could see them. As a PA "float," it was my job to commute to any of the company's twenty clinic locations in Dallas and Fort Worth when reinforcements were needed, and to see patients until the queue was empty.

Team dynamics and prescribing preferences differed considerably among the clinics, and I was expected to adjust my practices according to my de facto supervising physician for the day. Many of them left lasting impressions on me for their clinical acumen. Some were memorable for their personal quirks as well.

One physician, Dr. Eckert, had a reputation for being all business, all the time. She always pulled back her graying hair into a severe bun, and when she disapproved of something, her thin, unsmiling lips nearly disappeared into the permanent frown lines on her face. She was very particular about everything; it was her way or no way. She also had no qualms about attending to her personal grooming at the clinician workstation we shared.

I didn't think anything of it the first time she trimmed a few of her fingernails next to me. Our hands undergo quite a bit of trauma between washing, examining, and performing procedures. I didn't get manicures anymore because they rarely lasted more than two or three days.

"My god, every time I turn around, these guys need to be cut again," Dr. Eckert said as the emery board made an appearance. "I can't do a physical exam with talons."

I murmured absentmindedly in agreement. Technically, she was right, and our PA professors had told us the same thing many times. Long nails are uncomfortable for patients when we palpate their bare skin. More importantly, they can prevent us from obtaining pertinent information from the physical exam since we have sensation only in our finger pads.

On a subsequent shift with Dr. Eckert, I was speaking to a pharmacist over the phone and glanced down momentarily at the chart to confirm a patient's prescription. At that exact moment, a shard of nail fell across the page and obscured my handwriting. I looked up to see Dr. Eckert's foot just inches away, propped up on our workstation. She was cutting her toenails this time.

"Whoops, that one got away from me," she said, winking at me as she redirected the wayward clipping toward the small pile in front of her.

I drew my arm back with disgust and finished my call with the pharmacist, trying to ignore the steady clipping sounds that I was now aware of after that toenail visited my poor chart. *Eww.*

It turns out Dr. Eckert's usual clinic team had previously raised concerns about her pop-up nail salons. Management reviewed the situation and determined that Dr. Eckert saw an average of five and a half patients per hour, well above the company's physician benchmark of four per hour. So long as her personal activities did not affect her work product and patient safety, she was free to continue them. She always cleaned her workstation with Lysol afterward, and never cut her nails in areas with laboratory materials or food. Everyone else would just have to accept her grooming habits.

Another physician I worked with, Dr. Samuels, was very passionate about women's health. She was selected to speak on a panel at a local conference, and I listened with admiration as she shared her insights on topics ranging from bleeding during pregnancy to hot flashes during menopause. Someday, I hoped to communicate complicated information to my own patients with the same ease.

"It's wonderful to have so many options now to treat menopause symptoms," she said as the other speakers on the panel nodded in agreement. "Some of these women have been suffering for years with what they think are urinary tract infections. It changes everything when I tell them, 'I can prescribe you something different that you'll love for your coochie.'"

I almost choked on my coffee. *Did she just say 'coochie'?! To a patient?* I hadn't been a PA for that long, but I was absolutely certain that *coochie* wasn't the preferred term. Regardless of the informal language a patient might use when referencing her nether regions (*vag, clit, booty hole, hoo-ha, va-jay-jay, back door*), we had always been instructed to keep a straight face and respond using formal medical terms. Certainly, no scenario existed in which we initiated the mention of a patient's coochie.

Murmurs from the audience and raised eyebrows on one of the panel physician's faces confirmed that I wasn't the only one thrown off by this unscripted moment.

"Aaand that'll conclude the presentation portion; let's go to the Q&A," the moderator said hastily.

I worked only a few times with Dr. Noles, but I liked him immediately. His clinic was one of the busiest, and several emergencies often required his attention at the same time: one patient was bleeding, another was in the early stages of anaphylactic shock, yet another was suffering a heart attack. Dr. Noles always took the hectic unpredictability in stride. Even in situations when mere minutes could mean the difference between life and death, between consciousness and coma, he remained the picture of mental clarity and decisiveness.

"Hell no, I don't always feel calm," he said, laughing when I spoke of my admiration. "But I'll fake it till I make it; it's the only way I can be effective under pressure."

Dr. Noles advised me that a good sense of humor was also essential and had saved him and many of his urgent care colleagues from getting burned out. Indeed, I had often overheard him telling a dad joke to a worried patient. Afterwards, the latter seemed just a little more at ease. Dr. Noles often kidded around with the medical team, too, which made the clinic a more enjoyable place to work.

One evening, I slumped into my chair after we finished a doozy of a 10a to 10p shift. All eight exam rooms had been at full capacity all day, and the last patient had arrived right at 9:58 p.m. I was drained. Dr. Noles, on the other hand, was somehow operating at the same 10 out of 10 energy level that he had started with at 10 a.m.

"Emily, you need anything from me?" he asked cheerfully.

"No, I've got it, thank you! Almost done with my last chart," I said. He gave me a thumbs up.

"Great, then I'm gonna make like a fetus."

I stared at him, confused. "You're gonna what?"

In full seriousness, without even a hint of a smile, he answered, "Make like a fetus and head out."

Sadly, a few of my memories of physician colleagues are less lighthearted. I worked on occasion with Dr. Martin, who had been with the company for twenty years and was well respected for his bedside manner and solid clinical practices. The first time I saw him, he shook my hand warmly and thanked me for driving an hour and a half to help with the sudden influx of patients at his location. The last time I saw him, his hands hung limply by his sides as two security guards escorted him out of the clinic.

Stunned, I asked one of the nurses, Mandy, what happened. She confided in me that a few months prior, a patient had observed Dr. Martin nod off while he listened with his stethoscope. Quick thinking on Mandy's part convinced the patient that Dr. Martin liked to close his eyes so he could focus better on the heartbeat, almost like meditation.

"Did she buy it?" I asked. Mandy shrugged.

"Apparently, because she didn't file a formal complaint. And when I thought about it later, it's always possible that's actually what happened. Dr. Martin's really quiet when he's listening, and he probably did rest his eyes for a minute. The patient saw that and just freaked out."

"Did you ever ask him about it?"

"I didn't want him to feel embarrassed. None of us had ever seen him fall asleep at work. Anyway, everyone forgot about it after a while. Then last week, he called me into his office after work and asked me to have a drink with him."

My eyes widened; Dr. Martin was married. "What did you say?"

"I told him, 'Dr. Martin, I'm flattered, but I'm happily married.' He said he wasn't talking about going on a date or having an affair, just unwinding because it had been a crazy day . . . then he took out a bottle of Jack from his desk."

"What?! He had that at work? I hope he wasn't drinking when he was seeing patients."

Mandy shook her head. "Me too. I started wondering about that time the patient said he fell asleep . . . I just couldn't see it though. You know how Dr. Martin always does everything by the book. I told him my answer was still no and he said that was fine, he would just have a drink by himself."

For a time, Mandy vacillated about what to do. She really liked Dr. Martin—we all did—and she didn't want him to get in trouble. Ultimately, though, Mandy told her manager. She then had to awkwardly stand by as the manager questioned Dr. Martin about the alleged events. Dr. Martin admitted to keeping alcohol in his desk that day and offering Mandy a drink. But, he insisted, he always knew his limits and never had a single sip when patients were in the clinic. Apparently, it was against company policy for employees to consume alcohol on the premises, but not necessarily grounds for termination if the clinic was already closed for the night.

Dr. Martin then reluctantly allowed the manager to search his entire desk. In the topmost drawer, in the very back behind his signature stamp and business cards, was a second compartment filled with mini liquor bottles. Mandy's heart had sunk when they came into view, and Dr. Martin immediately started begging them both for compassion. He revealed that he had been struggling with alcohol for several months after he and his wife began having marital issues. Soon, he was bringing alcohol to work because he needed a drink before and after his shifts to function. He knew he had a problem, but he was too ashamed to tell anyone. His home life was crumbling because he spent all his time and energy at work; now he had lost control of his drinking, too. Going to a therapist for help was out of the question because he or she would be ethically and legally obligated to report it to the medical board. Every conceivable option would lead to the same outcome: he would lose his license to practice medicine, and with it, his reputation, his income, and his barely surviving marriage. Dr. Martin had thus chosen the only viable alternative he saw. He continued to show up on time every day for his patients, and for us, and hid his painful secret behind his office's closed doors.

I felt sick to my stomach upon hearing all that Dr. Martin had been dealing with, alone. I understood perfectly his responsibilities to the public as a physician, but he was first and foremost a human being. He needed compassion just as much as the patients he continued to care for. Like them, he also had a medical condition that required treatment and support. But fear of judgment from colleagues and friends, and of punishment from licensing boards, prevented his recovery. The very institution that decreed he should 'do no harm' had ironically made Dr. Martin terrified to get help, and therefore more likely to unintentionally harm a patient or himself. And like so many other healthcare professionals silenced by this same fear, he ended up losing everything, anyway.

Finally, there was Dr. Meyers, the physician who showed me I still had much to learn about my new place on the medical totem pole. An imposing woman with a temper as volatile as a pot of boiling water, Dr. Meyers believed people had no excuses when it came to reaching their full potential. She had wanted to become a doctor since age five, and had even signed her name as "The Future Dr. Amanda Meyers." As the first person in her family to graduate from college, she took all her roles—doctor, mother, wife, and sister—very seriously, and expected others to do the same.

One day, Dr. Meyers pulled me aside while I was chatting and laughing with a couple of nurses during a break. She gave me a withering look that instantly wiped the smile off my face, and I obediently planted my butt into the chair next to hers. The nurses raised their eyebrows at me as they slinked away; we all knew Dr. Meyers could go from quietly commanding to furiously screaming in a matter of minutes.

"Emily, you're a provider now. You're here to use your brain to take care of patients, not to be friends with the staff," she began sternly. "I'm not saying be mean to the nurses, but under no circumstances should you be chatting about what they or you do in your personal time outside of work. Then they're going to see you as an equal."

"I kind of feel like their equal," I admitted sheepishly. "They all have more experience than me, and I've learned a lot from them." This was an understatement; I felt like I owed my entire survival in the fast-paced world of urgent care to the nurses. From their feedback and willingness to share their skills, I learned how to anticipate patient questions, communicate instructions clearly at discharge, and perform various laboratory tests. I emulated the nurses' caring yet businesslike interactions with patients and took note of how they handled disgruntled or uncooperative ones. The nurses forgave me for my mistakes and kept me humble.

Dr. Meyers shook her head emphatically and straightened my crooked perspective of the medical hierarchy.

"It's fine to learn from them, but at this stage of your career when you're younger than most of them, they won't respect your authority as a PA if they see you as an equal. We're the ones ultimately responsible for the patient, and it's our licenses on the line if something bad happens. If staff doesn't take us seriously, it hurts our patients, it hurts us, it hurts everyone."

"Okay," I said uncertainly.

"You need to be intentional and create the boundary between personal and professional. They need to know that when Emily the PA says 'do this', they need to do it now and do it right. Do you understand what I'm saying?"

"Yes."

She nodded, satisfied. "Good. I'll be watching."

And with that, Dr. Meyers left me alone with my thoughts about what I had revealed to the nurses about my personal life (went out to dinner with my boyfriend that weekend). Personal and professional boundaries with patients had always been a no-brainer for me, but nurses and staff? How was I going to earn their respect when they knew I was still learning?

THE BIRDS AND THE BEES

A nurse handed me a clipboard on a busy afternoon in the clinic. "Eighteen-year-old just checked in for itchy eyelids," she summarized from the patient's intake form.

"Thanks, Rhonda," I replied distractedly as I took the clipboard in my outstretched hand. Patients were coming in like hotcakes. A case of itchy eyelids should be a quick appointment; it was probably the springtime allergies that plagued everyone in Texas. The patient had filled out the form in his own words in the waiting room, and I scanned it for all of ten seconds before whipping my chair around. Rhonda was already off triaging another patient somewhere.

"Did the patient fill this out, or are y'all messing with me?" I called to the other nurses nearby, waving the clipboard. They looked up, perplexed.

"What is it?" one asked, making her way over to me. I checked that there were no patients within earshot, then held the clipboard at arm's length and read aloud:

Describe your symptoms today:
Itchy and swollen eyelids. Kinda blurry in one.

What were you doing when you noticed your symptoms?
At home watching TV.

Where did the injury/incident/pain occur?
Idk.

Do you have any other symptoms?
Rash on my penise. Irritated a lil.

The nurses giggled and snorted like I had just performed a stand-up comedy routine.

"A lil! I would be more worried about that rash than your itchy eyelids!" one remarked.

"You don't know where the incident occurred? I can tell you the rash on your penis wasn't from watching TV!" another howled. "If you can't spell it, you shouldn't be using it."

I couldn't help laughing, too, and it took a few minutes to collect myself. *Maybe this wouldn't be just a quick visit for itchy eyelids after all.*

After I greeted the patient, I let him tell me in his own words what brought him into the clinic. I learned that "irritated a lil" referred to his itchy, swollen eyelids, which had been bothering him for several days. He had first noticed them while watching TV because the screen looked "kinda blurry." The rash on his penis had appeared just the night before, and he had added it under "other symptoms" because the intake form was designed for only one chief complaint. Unlike his eyelids, however, the rash was irritated *a lot.*

I suspected gonorrhea, a sexually transmitted infection (STI), upon hearing the classic symptoms of burning urination, penile discharge, and a rash after having sex without a condom. I called for Rhonda to come chaperone me. The young man had earned himself a urethral swab—a long Q-tip that I inserted into the opening of his penis and then rolled between my fingers to collect a sample of discharge for testing (at the time, urine tests for gonorrhea were not widely available yet). As the patient winced and cried out in protest, I seized the opportunity to urge him to use a condom every time he had sex in the future so that he would never need to go through this unpleasant process again.

"I already told the girl we're not gonna hang out anymore," he responded with a shrug as he zipped up his pants. Rhonda kept silent until we stepped out of the exam room.

"Hoo, Emily, I hope you swabbed him extra hard. You need to get him to wrap that thing up before he gets a disease he can't get rid of. My son would get an ass-whooping."

Rhonda summed up the fine line I walked with teenage patients precisely. Even though I was only a few years older than most of them, I needed to establish my authority as both the adult and the professional. But I wasn't a parent. If I came across as one, I was unlikely to gain their trust or influence their actions.

Once the young man was dressed, I changed tactics. I asked him what he knew about gonorrhea, other than how painful it currently felt, and he admitted that he'd never heard of it ("Is it like herpes or something?"). I did my best to be brief and use understandable terms, and I was pleased when his responses showed he was listening.

"For real?" he said, arching his eyebrows when I explained that a gonorrhea infection could cause infertility. "I don't want her to not be able to have babies."

"I know you don't," I replied gently. "You're a good guy. You can still tell her to get treated so it doesn't happen." He nodded.

"For sure. I'll call her later."

"And what about using a condom the next time you have sex?" I added. He hesitated before answering.

"I'll think about it. Having gonorrhea sucks. I'm just glad it's not forever, like HIV."

"You got lucky," I agreed. "Are you ready to get the shot?"

"Yeah."

I fetched Rhonda for a Rocephin injection. In cases like these, where we have high clinical suspicion of a disease based on the patient's history, exam, or both, we treat rather than wait to confirm the diagnosis. Test results from his swab could take up to a week to come back. The risk of side effects from the shot was minimal compared to the risks of infecting more sexual partners, suffering with continued symptoms, or contracting other STIs.

Would he use a condom next time? Probably not. But he had at least a little more perspective now on unprotected sex. I had demonstrated that I cared about what happened to him, that I wanted to protect him from diseases. And I'd done it without scolding or punishing him like a parent might. This was the art of "building rapport" that professors had instructed us on since day one of PA school. The relationship between a patient and a clinician was never automatic. We started off as complete strangers, and the clinician had to display respect and genuine concern to create trust. Only then could we apply our specialized knowledge and skillset to solve patients' problems and make them better. I loved the challenge. This was what I had gone through all the blood, sweat, and tears for. This was the joy of healing those who sought my help.

Ms. Jackson's chart showed that she had been to our urgent care clinic for the same chief complaint of "vaginal discharge and STI testing" multiple times. We had treated her twice for chlamydia, an STI that spreads just as easily as gonorrhea and can also cause infertility, pelvic pain, and life-threatening blood infections. Dr. Dorsanio had documented that he counseled Ms. Jackson on protection and pregnancy prevention methods.

Patient not interested in contraception, although she does not want to get pregnant, he had written in his last note.

When I opened the door, Ms. Jackson was standing off to the side and awkwardly holding the bottom half of her dress in a bunched-up heap around her waist. Her tan legs were exposed, almost up to her bikini line.

"Hi, Ms. Jackson," I said, concealing my surprise. "We're not doing an exam just yet . . . if you want to sit down first." She shook her head and continued to clutch the dress like a deflated inner tube.

"I can't sit down. I'm not even wearing underwear because it hurts," she said anxiously.

"Oh, okay," I responded awkwardly. "Tell me what's going on."

Ms. Jackson's present concerns were vaginal discharge and abdominal pain so uncomfortable that she could barely sit, walk, or sleep. After I asked the typical questions about what symptoms she had and how long they had been going on, I gathered her sexual history. By now, it was a practiced and almost mundane task for me, like gathering information about what a patient usually ate for breakfast. I phrased the series of questions the same way we had learned them in school.

"Are you sexually active?"

"Yes."

"Do you have sex with men, with women, or both?"

"*Men*, one hundred percent," she answered with a little laugh. I nodded and continued, "How many people have you had sex with in the last month?"

"Three." She hesitated. "But it's complicated."

With an air of professional disinterest, I replied, "That's okay, go ahead."

"Let's call them guys A, B, and C, okay? Guy A and me had sex a bunch of times, but we broke up. Guy B and me had sex just one time. Then Guy A tried to get back with me and we had sex again two weeks ago, but we're still broken up. Guy C is my man, who was in jail and just got out. We had sex last week, and then I got with Guy A a couple days ago."

"Okay. Let me make a couple of notes here," I replied, keeping a neutral expression.

After confirming a few more details, I performed an exam and some blood and urine tests. I ruled out pelvic inflammatory disease, a more serious condition that could cause Ms. Jackson's symptoms and that often resulted from STIs like gonorrhea and chlamydia. Her urine test, however, showed she did have a coinfection with both bacteria.

"You think it was A, B, or C who gave me this?" Ms. Jackson asked. "I really hope it's not my man, but I have this feeling he's been messing around since he got out."

"We probably won't know which guy it was, but we're going to make sure we give you treatment today and get you feeling better. We're going to treat all three of them, too, because we don't want the infection to spread back to you or to someone else," I explained.

Fortunately, Ms. Jackson was willing to call Guys A and B, and to threaten Guy C ("Doctor Emily says we're not gonna find out who did this, but if I find out you're sleeping around I'm gonna cut off your dick."). At my suggestion, she encouraged them to come to our clinic to be tested and treated that day. State health departments and primary care offices required appointments, which could take days or weeks. In that time, her sexual partners could spread whatever they had to more unsuspecting people. After I treated Ms. Jackson with a Rocephin shot and azithromycin pills, I thanked her for coming in to see me.

"You're taking control of your health by getting tested and treated right away," I told her.

She seemed surprised. "Everyone else just tells me to

use condoms or to stop screwing so many guys. I even bring condoms and tell them I want to use them, but they won't do it, or they take it off."

"Don't stop speaking up," I replied encouragingly. "It's your body; you don't have to take 'no' for an answer."

"Yeah, the last thing I need is another baby right now. Is there anything else I can use except condoms?"

I nodded emphatically. "Yes, there are lots of options. Remember, only condoms block infections like HIV, though." I thought for a moment. "You know what, there's an OB/GYN I want you to meet. She's great and can go over all the choices and help you decide what's best for you. I want you to look this over and take it with you when you go to see her." I gave Ms. Jackson an infographic with different contraception options.

Within three months, Ms. Jackson had an IUD implanted to prevent pregnancy and was telling sexual partners that they were either wearing a condom or they weren't getting any. She continued to see me for occasional STI screenings and, thankfully, the results were always negative. As someone of the same age, I became quite fond of her and was pleased to know that she was doing well. Her trust in me was responsible for our getting to this point, and I never took it for granted.

HOW TO BE A PROFESSIONAL

Mr. Goldberg complained of vomiting and diarrhea for two days. He gave me a choppy history about how "it's coming out of both ends" in between dry heaves over a blue emesis bag. It sounded like gastroenteritis, which is common, usually caused by a virus, and self-limited (goes away on its own without treatment). Although I was running late for my next patient, I could see how uncomfortable Mr. Goldberg was and wanted to give him some relief, even if just for the time that he was in our clinic. I leaned toward him as he hung his head over his knees.

"Mr. Goldberg, I'm going to find you something for nausea that you can take while you're here; is that okay? It's called Zofran."

He retched again, then lifted his head slightly. "I've taken it before."

"Did you have any side effects?"

"No. How long does it take to start working?"

"Twenty to thirty minutes, sometimes even sooner," I responded. "We also give Phenergan injections, but we require that someone drives you home after because it can make you drowsy or dizzy. Plus, once you go home, you can't give yourself the shots."

Mr. Goldberg shifted uncomfortably in his chair and held his stomach. "Okay. I'll try the Zofran."

Once I returned with the medicine, I explained how to administer it at home.

"You just peel back the foil wrapper, push the pill through, and put it on top of your tongue. It dissolves, so you don't need to take it with water. You can also put it under your tongue." I extended my hand toward him with the tiny white pill.

"Careful, it's really small," I advised.

Without warning, Mr. Goldberg lowered his head and licked the pill out of my palm. The trail of warm wetness he left wasn't even the worst part; it was the audible slurp as he did so. I snatched my hand back, startled.

"Mmm, I feel better already," he murmured creepily as he looked up and met my eyes.

"That was . . . very uncomfortable," I finally managed, my contaminated hand dangling awkwardly by my side as I quickly composed myself. I bade Mr. Goldberg goodbye and scrubbed my hands thoroughly at the sink, disheartened that I hadn't come up with a more substantive response. *Very uncomfortable?* If a stranger had done the same thing to me in public, I probably would have backhanded him and told him to get the hell away from me. What made Mr. Goldberg think he could do that? Afterward, I told a colleague about the exchange. He looked disgusted.

"You don't have to tolerate that," he exclaimed. "If a patient does something gross, tell them they're being completely inappropriate and that they don't need to be our patient anymore."

"I wish I had thought of that on the spot. I just froze," I admitted.

"It happens," my colleague said with a shrug. "You just have to remind them you're a professional. You have so many patients to see. Don't waste your time with ones who don't respect you."

Outside of work, too, plenty of people were finding out that I was a healthcare professional. Both friends and strangers would ask what I recommended for their allergies, or whether I thought the pain in their [insert body part here] was serious. The medical challenges people threw my way excited me. My answers as a student had been based largely on rote memorization and secondhand patient vignettes. Now, I realized with a little puff of pride that I'd seen enough patients to confidently answer people's questions from experience. I could nearly always think of a similar scenario and how to approach the problem because I had done it before in the workplace. It was kind of amazing how my job was applicable everywhere.

One weekend, I was over at a friend's house when her 70-year-old father attempted to stand up from his recliner, lost his balance, and fell. I instinctively jumped up from the couch and was beyond relieved when Mr. Bell stood up unassisted and confirmed that he did not hit his head. He had apparently cut himself on something, however; a stream of blood slid down his shin. He sank back into the recliner, and I pumped the handle on the side to elevate the footrest.

While my friend hurried to find some bandages, I applied pressure to Mr. Bell's wound with a clean kitchen towel. Deep, cherry-red blood soaked through the checkered pattern.

"Do you take any blood thinners, Mr. Bell?" I asked, concerned.

He smiled ruefully. "No. Apparently, I'm just a little clumsy. My slipper got hung when I stood up, and next thing I know, I just went down. Say, you're a doctor, right?"

"PA," I clarified gently. They'd drilled into our heads in school that under no circumstances were we to misrepresent ourselves as doctors. I moved the towel slightly and took a peek. There was a gash in his thin, translucent skin, but the bleeding had slowed.

"Well, I guess it's good I hurt myself when you were here," Mr. Bell quipped.

"Do you know if you're up to date on your tetanus shot?"

"Tetanus? It's probably been twenty years since I had one of those! I think I got the pneumonia one a few years back, though."

I hid a smile. "That's good. I don't want you to get pneumonia, either. But we need to get you updated on your tetanus so this doesn't get infected." I glanced up as my friend returned with a few Band-Aids.

"I couldn't find the first aid kit," she said apologetically. She handed me a sewing kit instead that looked like it had been through the ringer. The lid and a few needles were missing, and the remaining ones had rust on them. One had some sort of suspicious gooey yellow substance on it.

"This will do just fine," Mr. Bell said, indicating the pitiful sewing kit. "Go ahead and stitch me up, Emily, I trust you."

I shook my head. "Lucky for you, it's very shallow and we don't need stitches. See? It's already stopped bleeding. I'm going to rinse it out and bandage you up, okay?"

Mr. Bell nodded and leaned back in his chair. "Whatever you say. You're the doctor."

After I got Mr. Bell cleaned up, my friend promised to take him to his PCP to recheck the wound. Mr. Bell had some questions about the tetanus shot, so I explained just as I would to a clinic patient that it prevented tetanus bacteria from getting into a wound and causing lockjaw.

"Good deal. Thanks again for patching me up," Mr. Bell said, smiling.

"Oh, it was nothing," I replied with a wave of my hand. It was a good feeling, being able to help someone in a moment of need, even if that was basic first aid and vaccine counseling. Mr. Bell respected me and believed in my abilities, so much so that he had been prepared to let me use some rusty, goo-covered needles and no anesthesia to sew up his leg when he lived just down the street from a hospital with real sutures and real anesthesia.

At the same time, I couldn't help but feel somewhat relieved that his injury hadn't required homemade stitches. It would have been terrible to cause the nation's only case of tetanus that year.

One beautiful fall day, my husband, Matthew, and I arrived at a friend's backyard to grill and watch football. I was looking forward to a relaxing evening after a stressful week at work. I could just kick back and be myself around my favorite people. The universe, however, had other plans.

Jeff, the host, watched as I approached the patio table with an ice-cold beer in one hand and a burger piled high with all the fixings on a plate in the other. He was standing next to a guy I didn't recognize. As I set my plate down, Jeff jerked his head towards me and said, "Emily's a PA. She can probably tell you what it is."

"Hey, how's it going? I'm Emily," I said, smiling at the guy. My stomach growled in anticipation; the burger smelled amazing.

"Hey, I'm Brett," he replied. "You mind checking out this rash? I have no idea what it is, and it's been there for a week."

Reflexively, I heard myself say, "Sure, I'd be happy to." I had become a PA to help people, and here was a man asking for my help. Put my professional hat on.

Brett made his way over to the corner where I was sitting. He pulled the neckline of his T-shirt to the side, and I dutifully leaned in for a closer look at the exposed skin on his chest. I could barely make out the rash in the shade of the backyard, and his dark chest hair didn't help matters. I ran through a list of standard questions: no pre-existing skin conditions or similar rashes in the past, no pets, no medications, no new exposures, no recent bug bites, no symptoms suggestive of an infection? Brett answered no to all.

"It itches like crazy. Do you think I should be worried?" he asked, already looking beyond worried.

"It's good that it isn't spreading and that you haven't been feeling sick," I reassured him. "It might be some skin irritation from something you've come in contact with. I'm sorry I can't really say much. It's a little pink right there, but it's hard to see without the proper lighting."

Wrong answer. Brett promptly put one leg up on the empty chair next to me and pulled his shirt off over his head. I glanced over his shoulder and pleaded silently with my husband from across the backyard to come save me. If only. My man looked absolutely tickled as he took in the scene: some random (now shirtless) guy had commandeered the corner of the patio table where people were eating, and I had my face only inches away from his chest. My expression probably betrayed my hanger and frustration at my failed attempts to return to the juicy burger on my plate that had surely gone cold by now.

"You can touch it if you want. I don't think it's contagious or anything, it just itches," Brett said to me.

"No thanks," I said quickly. Some of my friends were staring now, so I added in a gentler tone, "I think it's a poison ivy rash. Oozing is pretty common, and I know it looks bad, but it'll dry up and crust over without leaving a scar as long as you don't scratch it. I would try ice packs and over-the-counter hydrocortisone cream."

"Thank you for looking at it," he responded as he reached for his shirt.

"No problem. If it gets worse at all, or doesn't get better after a couple days, you should see your primary care doctor. They know your medical history and can examine the rest of your skin or get a sample if needed."

Whoa. Did I just throw an informal "CYA" (cover your ass) in there like I was at work? All the signs in Brett's case pointed to a benign cause, and I had acted in good faith at this impromptu barbeque consultation. But it was always possible that the rash was something serious or that things would go south. Brett might not seek timely medical care because I'd told him it was nothing to worry about. The chances that he would sue me, a complete stranger? Probably zero. But the Texas Good Samaritan Act exists precisely because people who experience an accident or medical emergency sometimes sue bystanders (including healthcare professionals) if someone ends up getting hurt in the process, even if the bystanders attempted to help. Likewise, no matter how honorable a clinician's intentions or how justifiable the intervention, every clinician and clinic administrator knows that people sue. The CYA had been pure instinct. Apparently, I had been a PA long enough now to learn that one could never be too comfortable or give too many caveats.

I finally sat down to finish eating my much-anticipated burger. Now that the show was over, Matthew strolled up and slid into the empty seat next to me at the table.

"Hey girl," he said with a cheesy grin. "You think you can check out some rashes on my body? I need to take my shirt off so you can touch my abs."

FAMILY PRACTICE

I spent the next several years working in family medicine, where my role expanded from provider to primary care provider. The transition from student to PA had been challenging, but this learning curve was far steeper. In addition to treating acute patient concerns, I was now also responsible for preventing new health problems and for managing long-term conditions like high blood pressure, diabetes, depression, and heart disease. The familiar feelings of uncertainty and inexperience insidiously crept in once again.

"You'll be comfortable with the medical conditions once you see them enough times, and we see it all here," my new supervising physician, Dr. Sinclair, assured me. "Sometimes the harder part is figuring out a patient's personality so you can adjust your strategy and communication style. Every patient is different, but you'll start to see patterns."

I wasn't exactly sure what Dr. Sinclair meant by that. I knew relationships with patients would no longer be single, fleeting interactions after which I would never see them again, as they were in urgent care. That was the biggest appeal of primary care for me. I could learn my patients' stories, be involved in their journeys, and make a real difference in their lives.

Dr. Sinclair was a force of a man, and some days I could barely believe I was working in the same clinic as him. After growing up in rural Kentucky, he completed his training and family medicine residency at the University of Washington, one of the best programs in the country. He spent the next ten years working at federally-certified rural health clinics in several states, specifically those designated as medically underserved areas by the Health Resources and Services Administration (HRSA) because of "a shortage of primary care providers, a high infant mortality, high poverty, and/or a high elderly population." All HRSA clinics must employ at least one PA or NP, so Dr. Sinclair was comfortable working with midlevel clinicians and saw them as valuable in a team-based approach to care. He also traveled to train rural clinicians since they were often the sole healthcare resource for thousands of miles. All the while, he envisioned opening his own practice one day. At a medical conference in Houston, Dr. Sinclair met his future wife, a CPA who specialized in medical practice accounting. Within two years, they moved to Dallas, married, and started Sinclair Family Practice together.

In observing Dr. Sinclair, it was obvious how he had managed to build all of this and garner such an exceptional reputation in the greater Dallas area. Not only did he have shrewd powers of perception and intuition, but also an equanimity that I had rarely seen thus far in my career. Dr. Sinclair never acted in haste or alarm, always with purpose and confidence. He believed that a PCP should be the anchor for a patient's health, a reliable person to turn to both when feeling sick and feeling well. Dr. Sinclair vowed timely, accessible care for acutely ill patients, and sacrificed his personal time to offer evening and weekend appointments. He encouraged those with chronic conditions to come in for regular follow-ups, thereby allowing him to address any problems as they naturally arose. Whether he was listening to a patient, or to me, no detail escaped him, and no angle was overlooked. In a patient experience survey, one patient described Dr. Sinclair this way: "Pleasant, professional, thinks about problems before answering, offers alternatives. Discusses problems WITH you in a consultative approach." That was the essence of this great and humble man.

Before long, I began to see the vast range of personalities Dr. Sinclair had promised. I discovered that patients had a wide variety of approaches to and perspectives about health and medical care. There was never a dull moment.

Dr. Google

I turned the doorknob to an exam room one morning and was blasted with something positively foul. It smelled like a geyser had erupted inside, and my eyes immediately began watering. A woman with beach-blonde waves and a flowy pale-pink blouse was leafing through an old issue of *People Magazine*, while a cute toddler played quietly with a Hot Wheels car at her feet. They both looked up as I entered.

"Hi, Sammy, hi, Ms. Brenton. What brings you in today?" I smiled at the mother while avoiding breathing through my nose. I saw nothing to explain the stench.

"Sammy's been having diarrhea for two days, and I think it's *C. diff*," Ms. Brenton replied anxiously. She didn't break eye contact as Sammy drove his car over her black, pointy-toed flats and up her shin with an enthusiastic *vroom*.

"Has Sammy had *C. diff* before?" I asked. Short for *Clostridium difficile*, *C. diff* is a bacterium that can cause severe inflammation of the large intestine.

Ms. Brenton shook her head. "No, but I googled it, and I'm sure that's what it is. I think he might need to be hospitalized."

Uh oh, Dr. Google. I'd seen patients get themselves all worked up after searching a common and nondescript symptom online, which inevitably turned into a possible diagnosis of cancer or imminent death. A worried mother and Dr. Google seemed like a particularly dangerous combination.

"Okay, why don't we start at the beginning so I can get the

full story," I said, gently steering Ms. Brenton toward a medically sound diagnosis. "Has he had a fever?"

"No, no fever."

"And has he been eating, sleeping, and playing like normal?"

She hesitated. "For the most part. He threw up once at the beginning, but he's sleeping fine, and his appetite's been good. He had his cereal and juice this morning."

I nodded. I had been silently observing Sammy for any signs of dehydration like blue skin, lethargy, or lack of tear production. He was energetic and looked happy as a clam as he scrambled up and down from Ms. Brenton's lap like she was a jungle gym. His hair was the same brilliant blonde. A lock of it fell over his eye, and he smiled shyly when he caught me looking at him.

Ms. Brenton had been carefully counting Sammy's soiled diapers and reported three episodes of diarrhea a day. Soft, sometimes watery, but no blood or mucus.

"And he hasn't taken antibiotics or acid reflux medicines recently?"

"No."

I smiled reassuringly. "Well, good news: his symptoms aren't consistent with diarrhea caused by a *C. diff* infection. I think it's a virus. Let's take a look at your belly, Sammy."

I listened to Sammy's bowel sounds and palpated his abdomen, which resulted in quite a few giggles but no expressions of pain. I let him play with my stethoscope as I reiterated my diagnosis to Ms. Brenton.

"I looked through, like, fifty images on Google!" she protested shrilly. "His poop looked just like the pictures—let me show you." She leaned over and reached into her purse. I thought she was going for her cell phone. Instead, she pulled out a diaper that was barely sealed and sagged with about a pound of poo. It took everything for me not to gag as the foul smell in the room increased exponentially. How had other patients been able to stand it in the waiting room?

"Please wrap that up and put it in the trash—the red biohazard one," I mouth-breathed. Ms. Brenton looked offended, and I added placatingly, "It was a good thought, but diarrhea infections can be very contagious, so we don't want them to spread from the poop to other people in the clinic."

After she disposed of the diaper and I had sufficiently recovered from the putrid odor, I explained that Sammy's diarrhea was likely due to Norovirus, the most common cause of gastroenteritis. Sammy didn't need hospitalization, but I reviewed signs of dehydration and other red flags should the situation change. Hydration, bland foods, and careful handwashing before eating or drinking should otherwise take care of his symptoms in the next couple of days. Ms. Brenton looked relieved and bounced Sammy on her lap.

"Thank you. Those pictures and horror stories online really freaked me out," she admitted.

I nodded emphatically. "I tell all my patients, 'Beware Dr. Google.' Anyone can post medical stuff online, and I see inaccurate and misleading information all the time. You can make yourself sick just worrying that you have a tumor or some rare disease."

"Dr. Google, ha! I like that," Ms. Brenton said with a laugh as we stood up to say goodbye.

Later, I told my good friend, a pediatrician, about the unexpected poop sample that was presented to me as evidence of *C. diff*. She laughed knowingly ("Moms bring me their kids' diapers after a blowout or show me dirty tissues full of snot every other day") and went to the cupboard.

"I have another one of these on my desk at work," she told me, returning with a mug. I looked closely: *Please do not confuse your Google search with my medical degree.*

A 52-year-old patient named Mr. Cox harnessed the powers of his Google search in a more surprising way. During grappling—a fighting technique in jiu jitsu—Mr. Cox had experienced sudden, severe pain in his elbow and limited range of motion. An x-ray confirmed a posterior elbow fracture. I stretched an elastic sleeve called a stockinette over his muscular arm and fashioned a long splint with padding and wet plaster along it all the way to his bicep. I also referred Mr. Cox to an orthopedic specialist to ensure proper healing and, if necessary, to provide further intervention.

I accompanied Mr. Cox to checkout and had just turned to walk away when I overheard his conversation with the staff.

"Your total for today is $68. That's for the x-ray and the cast," the receptionist said.

"I'm not paying that," came the reply. I turned, surprised. Mr. Cox had been very pleasant during the appointment and seemed like a nice guy in general. I'd already informed him of the cost for the procedures before we went through with them.

"I'm sorry, sir, it's just the portion you're responsible for because you haven't met your insurance deductible yet," the receptionist said patiently.

"But I didn't get anything out of the appointment," Mr. Cox declared.

"You . . . didn't have that cast on when you came in, sir." The receptionist hesitantly pointed to the splint, and Mr. Cox responded by folding his hands across his chest, as if that would make it disappear. He wasn't giving in.

"Yeah, but why do I need to pay you guys $68 to tell me my elbow's broken and that I need a splint? Google already told me that for free!"

Dr. Google had struck again.

Can Anxiety Kill You?

While it's normal to worry about things from time to time, I learned from one woman's story the unfortunate costs of excessive anxiety or misguided concerns. One afternoon, Dr. Sinclair beckoned me to his office after coming out of a patient room.

"I need to tell you about this young woman: Ms. Richards. You might be seeing her for follow-up after she gets out of the hospital," he said, pushing her chart toward me across the desk. He directed my attention to Ms. Richards' medication allergy list, which included several different antibiotics: amoxicillin, sulfa, ceftriaxone, levofloxacin, and metronidazole. Recorded reactions consisted of abdominal cramps, nausea, diarrhea, and yeast infection, among others.

"That's an impressive list for a twenty-year-old," I mused with raised eyebrows.

Dr. Sinclair grunted. "That's because she probably isn't allergic to most of them; her reactions are just common side effects of almost every antibiotic." He tapped a spot on the chart. "Maybe sulfa drugs, because she had 'hives and wheezing' with those, but she refuses to let me prescribe antibiotics in any of these classes."

"But that's, like, most of the antibiotics we prescribe!" I exclaimed.

"Exactly." He leaned forward confidentially and added, "I'm going to let you in on a little secret. If a patient says they have ten or more medication allergies, your antennae should be up for a psych patient." He nodded sagely, as if he had just imparted the solution to modern medicine's most elusive mystery.

"What do you mean?" I asked.

"I mean, they're scared to take medications, worried about side effects, or just anxious about everything. Ms. Richards is convinced that the side effects she has are allergies, and doesn't realize she's putting herself in danger by not taking an antibiotic. She had a simple UTI last week, and her culture showed it wasn't resistant to anything."

"She wouldn't take Macrobid? She's not allergic to that," I pointed out.

"No, she was so sure she'd have a reaction to that, too, even though it's in an entirely different class. There was nothing I could do to talk her out of it. She decided to take nothing. The infection spread, and now she has sepsis."

"Oh my gosh," I said, alarmed. Sepsis is a life-threatening medical emergency caused by an underlying infection. Without antibiotics, sepsis leads to organ failure, shock, and death.

Dr. Sinclair nodded grimly. "I told her up front before I sent her to the hospital, that this isn't the time to refuse antibiotics because she won't survive without them."

"What if she goes into septic shock?" I asked quietly. "Can they give her antibiotics if she says she's allergic?"

"They always weigh risk versus benefit. If the risk of her taking the antibiotics is possible diarrhea or a yeast infection, but the risk of not taking them is death . . . She's only twenty years old. They're going to do everything they can to save her life."

Dr. Sinclair closed the chart, dispirited, and we sat in silence for a moment. Even though I had never met Ms. Richards, I felt Dr. Sinclair's frustration, his incomprehension of how she could be so unyielding that she put herself in harm's way. What I didn't expect was the look of helplessness in his eyes. Why would patients come to us in times of need if they were going to reject our medical advice? Why wouldn't they let us help them while we still could?

Ms. Richards was admitted to the ICU shortly after that conversation. I never saw her for a hospital follow-up visit; she died a week later.

The Embarrassed Patient

A 29-year-old woman named Ms. Ritter had been dealing with vaginal discharge for nearly three weeks. Originally white in color, the discharge had progressively become milky green, thick, and associated with itching and burning. An embarrassing smell had also developed "down there." It had gotten so bad that she was afraid her coworkers would notice, and she had started changing her underwear several times throughout the workday.

I assured Ms. Ritter that her symptoms were common; many things could disrupt the normal vaginal environment. I asked a few questions to narrow down the possibilities: Had she taken a bubble bath or used a douche? Had she taken any antibiotics? Had she recently had sex? Ms. Ritter said that she had last been sexually active over a month ago with a male partner and had used protection, and she didn't know if he had any symptoms. Bacterial vaginosis and trichomoniasis vaginalis were at the top of my differential, especially because of the odor and color she described.

Ms. Ritter removed her underwear for the exam. As soon as I pushed back the privacy drape covering her lap, my face was in the direct line of fire. She hadn't been exaggerating about the stench; it smelled like an animal had crawled inside her and was rotting away. While she apologized profusely, I remained professional, telling her not to worry while I focused on my exam. I parted the labia and guided a speculum past copious discharge to better visualize the vagina and cervix.

A small, cylindrical object eventually came into view. Using sponge forceps, I slowly drew it out, careful not to leave any part behind. I held up the putrid and almost unrecognizable culprit for Ms. Ritter to see. It was a tampon.

"Oh my god," she exclaimed, clapping a hand over her mouth in horror. "The last time I used a tampon was almost a month ago! My period's about to start again."

"The important thing is, it's out now, and the source of the infection is gone," I said matter-of-factly. As I helped her out of the stirrups and into a seated position, I asked about symptoms associated with toxic shock syndrome, the potentially fatal condition that every box of tampons warns about. Fortunately, Ms. Ritter hadn't had headaches, vomiting, diarrhea, or rashes, and her vital signs were normal.

"Good. Then you won't need any antibiotics," I responded. "The discharge should go away on its own, and I want you to wash the area only with warm water. And maybe stick to pads for your next period?"

Ms. Ritter nodded her head vigorously. "Oh, I will! I'm never wearing a tampon again in my life!"

I left her to get dressed. Just another vaginal discharge mystery, solved.

Sirens sounded outside the clinic one afternoon. A tornado warning. Moments later, the power went out, and as the clinic plunged into darkness, so did the note I had just typed for my last patient of the day. Swallowing my despair, I prayed autosave would come through for me.

A flurry of activity followed: doors opened and shut, and several voices swelled in volume, talking over each other. I fumbled in my desk drawer for my cell phone and turned the flashlight on to see Dr. Sinclair emerge from a patient room.

"Perfect timing," he said sarcastically. "Will you bring your flashlight in here so I can finish the exam on this young man? I tried to use mine, but I couldn't get the right angle with one hand."

"Sure, no problem." I followed behind him with the flashlight. The exam room was pitch-black because there were no windows.

"Sorry about that, Mr. Gaines. I've got some light now," Dr. Sinclair said in the darkness to my right.

I raised my phone to locate Mr. Gaines, and all I could see in the beam of light was a penis.

I let out a startled gasp, then scrambled for something

professional to do or say to cover up my reaction. I don't know who was more mortified, me or the patient. He quickly bent down to grab his shorts from around his ankles, but they got caught on his shoes, so he gave up and just clapped his hands over his crotch. Meanwhile, I stammered something along the lines of "sorry for surprising you; I'm just here to provide the lighting," and frantically redirected the light toward the ceiling.

Dr. Sinclair seemed oblivious to what had just transpired.

"Alright, Mr. Gaines, let's try this again. I'm going to have you turn your head and cough so I can check for a hernia. Emily's going to hold the light so I can see what I'm doing."

After Dr. Sinclair pronounced Mr. Gaines hernia-free, the latter pulled up his shorts at warp speed, and I apologized once more for catching him by surprise. Once Dr. Sinclair and I stepped outside, I swung around.

"You didn't tell him I was coming in?" I cried.

"No, I just told him I needed more light and I'd be back once I found one," Dr. Sinclair said, laughing. "I didn't know he was just going to stand there butt naked, waiting."

The Skeptical Patient

One afternoon, I entered the room to find a 10-year-old girl dressed in her school uniform on the exam table. Her mother was on a conference call at the foot of the bed, toggling the mute button on and off on her cell phone to talk to me.

"Carrie keeps saying her head itches, and I don't know if she's allergic to her shampoo or just has a dry scalp," the mother said.

"And it's been two weeks now?" I asked, donning examination gloves.

"Yes, two weeks. Hey, I'm at the doctor's office right now," she said loudly into her phone. "Angie can take you through last month's reports, and I'll jump in when I can."

I busied myself with inspecting the skin on Carrie's face and along her hairline. A row of swollen, pink welts dotted the nape of her neck.

"Are these itchy?" I asked, lightly running my fingers over them to confirm that they were raised. Carrie responded by scratching furiously at them for a moment.

As I separated the strands of her dark hair, looking for scalp redness or irregularity, a tiny gleaming version of what looked like a droplet of fish oil caught my eye. I tried unsuccessfully to remove the bead from Carrie's hair with my fingers.

"It looks like we have a nit, Mom," I said, lifting the strand of hair. "This is an egg, and that means we're dealing with lice."

Carrie's mother leaned closer and looked at the bead skeptically before pressing mute again on her phone.

"How can she have lice?" she asked as Angie's voice droned on about this quarter's gains next to us. "I wash her hair every day. That's probably just a piece of dandruff."

I started to explain how having lice doesn't mean someone has dirty hair when a little black louse walked along the piece I was holding.

"Oh, here's a live one!" I cried. I attempted to capture it between my thumb and pointer finger. I missed, and the louse fell onto Carrie's mother's shirt just as she unmuted herself to add her thoughts to Angie's presentation.

Carrie watched in amusement as her mother shrieked and swatted hysterically at her silk blouse. Her cell phone clattered to the floor while I sprayed the louse with Lysol and balled it up in the exam table paper.

"… Lindsay?" A concerned voice floated up from our feet over speakerphone.

"I have to go," Carrie's mother responded, flustered. She fumbled with her phone before taking a seat again. At last, I had her undivided attention.

"I'm prescribing an antiparasitic treatment for Carrie

called Nix," I explained once she'd composed herself. "I want you to wash her hair with her normal shampoo first. Put the Nix all over the scalp while her hair's still damp, then let it sit for ten minutes."

Carrie's mother assented, before thoughtfully saying, "Actually, my head has been itching a little this week, now that I think of it."

I promptly prescribed antiparasitic treatment for both mother and daughter. I reassured them that head lice was not from poor hygiene or dirty living conditions; it was quite common and nothing to be ashamed of.

When I called a week later to make sure treatment had been successful, Carrie's mother answered the phone.

"We followed your directions with the Nix, and we haven't had any more itching," she confirmed.

"Wonderful. Do you have any other questions for me?"

"No. I really appreciate your taking care of both of us, Emily. I shouldn't have doubted you; you know what you're doing."

And after that memorable appointment, she became one of my most loyal patients.

Another "buggy" encounter took an entirely different turn. A 40-year-old woman, Ms. Johnson, scheduled a consultation for an extensive rash that she had been to "four or five dermatologists for" but no one could figure out. The rash itched constantly and kept her awake at night. Red scratch marks and a few shallow ulcers covered her arms and legs. I inspected her hands and the webs between her fingers first—favorite sites of the mites that cause scabies.

"Have you found anything that makes the itching better?" I asked her.

"I spread mayonnaise on my skin," she replied. She lowered

her voice confidentially and added, "Then the bugs start to come out."

"Bugs?"

"Yes. They come out of my pores because they can't breathe through the mayonnaise."

"I see," I said slowly. "What do the bugs look like?"

Ms. Johnson enthusiastically described them: some were small and the shape of sunflower seeds, while others were stringy and worm-like. She had seen a bug come out of every pore of her body at some point in the last year.

"They get inside me when I'm asleep," she explained.

"Is anyone else at home itching or dealing with a rash, too?" The answer would be a key clue as to whether I was looking at an infestation of some sort.

"No, thank god. My son is good and my husband sleeps in the same bed as me, and he's fine. I'm the only one with the bites."

Oh boy. I was quickly realizing that the unknown cause of Ms. Johnson's rash was unlikely to be something rare that the dermatologists hadn't identified yet. I had an uneasy feeling in the pit of my stomach, but I covered my bases and suggested that she call an exterminator to inspect her house. Bed bugs and other pests are legitimate health hazards and can be difficult to treat. Sometimes, small bites on the skin or itching are the only evidence they leave behind. Ms. Johnson shook her head at my suggestion.

"All the doctors keep telling me that." She scrunched up her face and put on a sarcastic voice: "Get the pest control people to fumigate the house!" Then, with an annoyed sigh: "My family and I think I need to get the rash and itching under control first." She scratched her scalp absentmindedly for a moment, then used her fingers to smooth a Band-Aid on her right temple.

"What happened here?" I indicated the Band-Aid.

"When my head itches, sometimes I use a knife in there—"

I gaped. "In your head?"

"Uh huh, in my head, and I cut the skin open, and a bug comes out."

I finally sat down on the exam room stool and stared at the Band-Aid, dumbfounded. I had desperately hoped that my initial suspicions were wrong, but the diagnosis was indisputable. Ms. Johnson displayed classic symptoms of delusional parasitosis, a fixed, false belief that she was infested by parasites. She had brought a thick stack of negative test results from skin biopsies, blood tests, and the "bugs" (pieces of lint, dirt, scabs, etc.) as proof of the infestation. Various allergy and antiparasitic treatments had failed to help. I now had the added worry that she cut her own skin open and was operating on very little sleep. Self-mutilation and insomnia are both common with this condition, and their potential consequences are far more dangerous than just an itchy rash.

Antipsychotic medications can successfully treat delusional parasitosis, but I had to tread carefully. Several specialists had already reassured Ms. Johnson that there were no parasites. I wondered what alternative diagnoses they had offered to explain her symptoms. Her recollection was that "they just said they didn't know what it was." If I tried to convince her that this wasn't the work of bugs, she would simply seek out another clinician's opinion. If I suggested a psychiatrist for antipsychotic treatment, she might hear that I had called her crazy instead and refuse care. To help Ms. Johnson, I had to demonstrate empathy and trust. I needed to show that I believed her on some level. If not about the bugs, then at least about the distress her symptoms caused her. I agonized over the potential ramifications of each word before I spoke next.

"I can see that this rash is really stressing you out. I have some ideas, but I want to be realistic with you."

"Okay..." Ms. Johnson narrowed her eyes suspiciously but waited to hear me out.

"You've had this for a long time, so I think it's going to take a while for it to completely get better, even after we start treatment. I don't want you to give up after a few days because you're still itching. It can take several weeks for the medicine to reach its peak strength, but you'll know it's working because the itching will get a little better each week."

"I'll do anything—I'm desperate," Ms. Johnson insisted. Indeed, she looked close to tears.

"I can't even imagine. I want to focus today on the symptoms that are bothering you most and tackle those first."

Ms. Johnson told me the itching and insomnia were intolerable, and admitted to feeling increasingly depressed and helpless about the "infestation." I prescribed treatment to rebuild the skin barrier, reduce itching, and help her sleep. She, in turn, agreed to avoid scratching and cutting her skin, which I explained could worsen the itching, leave permanent scars, and cause infection or dangerous bleeding. I scheduled a follow up appointment to recheck her skin and review her medications in two weeks. With her consent, I also referred her to a psychiatrist for depression; this was my "in" to possible antipsychotic treatment. I watched Ms. Johnson leave, clutching her binder of test results representing hundreds of dollars' worth of investigation.

They had always told us in PA school that our medical knowledge, well-thought-out questions, and physical exam skills would lead us to the correct diagnosis and treatment. In reality, medicine was hardly ever that cut-and-dry. I knew exactly what this woman's diagnosis was and what she needed—but I wasn't sure if she'd ever get it. Making her better would involve more strategy than knowledge, something I hadn't considered before. I was going to have to live with the fact that, despite everything I knew about medicine, I couldn't cure all my patients. I might not even be able to help them.

Before I go any further, let me say that most of the patients I encountered at Sinclair Family Practice were wonderful. Honest, kind, and friendly, they were what we described in progress notes as "pleasant." Regrettably, the few who are not are often far more memorable. We recognize their names out of the thousands of patients we see, sometimes even when we've never met them. At best, they test our humanity. At worst, they make us question whether medicine is our true calling. As one of my colleagues put it, "It's the one percent that takes up ninety-nine percent of your time and energy."

Impatient Patients

My first patient on a Monday morning checked in for "flu-like symptoms." The nurse took her vitals and brought her straight back to one of my exam rooms, as there was no wait. After getting a history and noting a dry cough and considerable redness of her throat, I suspected the patient did in fact have the flu. I swabbed her nose for the virus and set the clinic laboratory's timer for ten minutes.

Not even three minutes had passed when the patient burst out of the exam room. I looked up from my computer, where I was reviewing the next patient's chart.

"Is everything okay, Ms. Hollis?" I asked, standing up.

"How much longer is it going to take to get my results?" she demanded.

"The rapid test takes ten minutes," I reminded her as I walked over. I was surprised that she sounded so annoyed when she hadn't been in the clinic for more than ten minutes total at this point. I knew she wasn't feeling well, though. I, too, could be cranky when I was sick.

Ms. Hollis' eyebrows shot up like I had just said the test would take an hour. "Ten minutes! I don't have ten minutes! What's the point of me waiting for the results?!" A few drops of her spit landed on my cheek, and I kept my voice steady as I wiped them away with the back of my hand.

"If the test is positive for the flu, you're still within the window for me to prescribe Tamiflu, as I mentioned. It can shorten your symptoms by a few days," I said. *I probably need a prescription myself,* I thought, picturing the invisible infectious particles from my cheek entering my airways.

Ms. Hollis did not like my answer. She grabbed her purse from the exam room and stormed to the front desk to demand a refund.

"If I wanted to wait ten minutes for a test result, I would have taken the rest of the morning off from work! I have a meeting in an hour, and it takes thirty minutes just to get back!"

I couldn't believe what I was hearing. The patient did realize *she* had scheduled this appointment, right? Surely, she could change the time of either her appointment or her meeting. Besides, I'd already explained what the test entailed and how long it would take for the results.

But the customer is always right, they say. Bonnie, the receptionist, politely issued Ms. Hollis a refund and apologized that she did not have a good experience. Ms. Hollis did not say another word as she slammed the door on her way out. Just seconds later, the lab timer went off and her test showed positive for the flu. I told Bonnie the verdict.

"You think she still wants to know if she has the flu?" she asked with a smirk.

I snorted. "Nah, she doesn't have time for that."

Jessica, another of our clinic's schedulers, approached me in the hallway one afternoon with a look of desperation.

"Mr. Stanley is giving us a hard time. He wants to see you for a travel consult and vaccines, but he doesn't have an appointment," she said in a low voice.

"And you told him we don't take walk-ins?" I asked as we headed for her desk.

"Yeah, I told him—and he knows. He's been a patient for ten years! He always comes swaggering in here like he's a celebrity. I even heard him tell other patients once that he's a 'priority patient,' which is total BS."

"What's a priority patient?" I repeated blankly.

Jessica put her hands on her hips, exasperated. "There's no such thing; it's something he made up. But then patients ask me how they get to be priority patients!"

"Oh Lord. Let me go and talk to him." This was the last thing I wanted to do, but it was a clinician's job to resolve patient conflicts. Jessica put a hand on my arm.

"Administration won't let us turn him away because he donates a lot of money to the clinic," she warned.

"What, so we're supposed to just drop everything and bend over backwards for him? That's ridiculous! He needs to follow the same rules as all the other patients."

"Oh no." Jessica suddenly looked at the screen like she had gotten bad news. I leaned over her shoulder as she refreshed the schedule: one of my patients had canceled her appointment for later that afternoon, and Mr. Stanley's name had replaced hers on the list. I'm assuming it was a coincidence and not because Mr. Stanley paid someone off, but either way, I hated that this guy was getting what he wanted. I had not become a PA to take care of only the richest patients. Healthcare was so inequitable already, and my duty was to recognize and help remove barriers. It was the people who had less—less money, less social support, less access to transportation and hospitals— who suffered the worst health consequences. If anyone should be prioritized, it was them, not this man who could afford any treatment, regardless of the cost.

Unfortunately, I couldn't turn a patient away if an appointment was available. When I entered the exam room that afternoon, I saw this 63-year-old hotshot donor in the flesh. Mr. Stanley was pacing, talking on speakerphone at an ungodly volume, and making no attempt to hang up when I greeted him. Instead, he held up his index finger.

"One second," he said to me, and then, to his phone, "Go ahead, Brad, you were saying?" I stared at him in disbelief as he resumed his conversation. This man wanted *me* to wait after he showed up without an appointment and we granted him the privilege of timely treatment? No, he wasn't going to disrespect me, my staff, or other patients like this. No one earns the right to healthcare or deserves better healthcare than anyone else. I didn't care how much money he had given to our clinic.

My professional facial muscles did their job and remained neutral. My voice, however, was stern.

"I'll come back when I'm ready for you," I said, loudly enough for both Mr. Stanley and Brad to hear. Then, I turned on my heel and walked back through the door. Although he later apologized for asking me to wait, Mr. Stanley evidently only did so to temporarily get into my good graces. It was far from the last time he pulled out his imaginary priority patient card.

Another patient also flaunted her status in attempts to get preferential care. Our clinic offered allergy shots twice a week for patients with designated immunotherapy orders from an allergist. To increase equal access to care, shot clinic was first-come first-served, irrespective of health insurance status or the ability to pay. A national allergy organization and a pharmaceutical company had partnered in this endeavor, and our patients were generally very grateful. Allergies in Texas can be brutal.

About ten patients waited in line on this particular day. The nurse greeted a patient at the front of the line and held the waiting room door open while they made friendly small talk. As the door closed behind them, a woman suddenly rushed towards it and called out, "Wait!"

I glanced up from my desk, which had a direct view of the waiting room door. The woman had managed to wedge her gigantic purse into it and keep it ajar. The nurse turned, surprised.

"Can I help you?" she asked.

"I'm Dr. Brewer, Becky's patient. I need to go next; I can't wait today," the woman said breathlessly. She glanced at the other patients in line, then unconvincingly added, "Sorry."

The nurse regarded Dr. Brewer with slight amusement before responding.

"With all due respect, doctor, that's not how we operate here. This is a first-come, first-served clinic. Everyone is here for their allergy shots, and they have to get back to work, too. If you don't have time today, you'll need to come back next week."

Dr. Brewer looked offended and craned her neck over the nurse's shoulder. "Is Becky here today? She can probably find a way to squeeze me in."

The nurse frowned. "Dr. Whelan's with another patient right now, so if you don't mind, I need to bring this young lady back. She's been patiently waiting while you and I have been having this conversation. If you could please get in line, that'll help everyone."

"Please just check with her," Dr. Brewer insisted before reluctantly trudging to the back of the line.

I raised my eyebrows, amazed at Dr. Brewer's persistence, and went back to my paperwork. Five minutes later, Dr. Whelan herself swept past me toward the waiting room. In front of all the other patients, Dr. Whelan advised Dr. Brewer that she was going to have to wait in line, no exceptions. That was the whole purpose of the clinic.

"You take care of patients. You know better than anyone else that this perpetuates unequal treatment," Dr. Whelan said flatly. "We can't use the initials on our white coats as black cards."

After she picked her jaw up off the floor, Dr. Brewer snapped, "This is ridiculous," and strode out of the clinic in a huff. Dr. Whelan watched her go and let out a heavy sigh before returning to her office. I realized that I, too, had been holding my breath. Bless her for doing the hard thing, the uncomfortable thing, for the good of her patients. I don't know if I'd have it in me to stand up to a physician that way.

Manipulating the System

A colleague collapsed into his chair next to me one day and started furiously banging a note out on his keyboard.

"You okay, Steve?" I asked him gently.

"These requests for emotional support animals are getting out of hand," he responded through clenched teeth.

"You had another one?"

"Yeah, and this lady's dog bit one of the temps who's covering for Julie."

My eyes grew wide. "What! Oh my god, are they okay?"

"I mean, the dog barely missed his jugular, and two patients had to pry its mouth open off his collarbone, but the man's alive." Steve clacked away on the keys as he spoke. "It had a 'service dog' vest on, but no service dog acts like that. And then the patient yells at *me* because I wouldn't write a letter for him as an emotional support pet. Your dog almost killed a person, lady!"

"I can't believe that happened," I said, horrified. "You told Joanna already?" Joanna was our clinic manager.

"Yeah. She told the patient she couldn't bring her dog to the clinic anymore for our employees' safety. The patient said we were discriminating against people with disabilities because he was a service dog and helped her with her anxiety." Steve shook his head in disbelief. "I'm sure he gave everyone else anxiety when that guy was screaming bloody murder."

He looked at me thoughtfully for a moment, then typed *nurse at risk for PTSD* into the encounter note describing the incident.

Later that morning, Joanna gathered all of us and briefly updated us on the gruesome attack. The nurse temp was in critical condition and undergoing emergency surgery on his jaw and collarbone. The clinic had offered to assist with his worker's comp claim. Joanna had also instructed the front desk staff to call security if a similar situation arose in the future. She encouraged the rest of us to stay watchful so that no unauthorized person sneaked through the locked clinic door.

I was distracted and on edge for the rest of the day, even though I hadn't witnessed the attack and nothing else crazy happened. The generic letters we occasionally provided in support of patients' dogs or cats had seemed harmless. But now this man, who had covered for Julie so she could take a vacation, was going to wake up from surgery and be emotionally and physically scarred. It was bewildering, all these things we did as clinicians that were never once mentioned during our training. How did a PA for humans even have the authority to decide if an animal benefited a patient?

Fortunately, our clinic's policy changed shortly thereafter. Patients would need to see their psychiatrists or their pets' veterinarians for any request involving animals. We would allow certified service dogs only, and we could still ask them to leave if they displayed aggressive behavior.

Then a patient brought a "ghost" service dog to an appointment for back pain. Ms. Clark arrived in a wheelchair, and I overheard her refusing to let Leila, the nurse, measure her weight because she couldn't stand up. Leila politely offered to assist her, but again, Ms. Clark refused.

Her appointment with me started normally enough. Ms. Clark was pleasant, and we made small talk about the 105 degree weather in Dallas, or as she called it, "Satan's Sauna." I asked her about her back symptoms and current ability to do various activities like get out of bed, dress, cook, and bathe. Within minutes, I had a gut feeling that something wasn't quite right. Ms. Clark's story was inconsistent, and she was what we referred to in medicine as a "poor historian": a patient who cannot remember or clearly articulate symptoms and health details. Clinicians base their differential on these details, broadening or narrowing the possible diagnoses appropriately. A cohesive clinical history effectively guides testing and treatment.

Ms. Clark also insisted on referring to me as "sweetheart."

"I would appreciate it if you would call me Emily; that's my name," I'd remind her politely. I needed to establish a minimal level of authority and respect, but I still wanted a good patient-clinician relationship.

"Emily, that's a nice name," Ms. Clark would respond thoughtfully. Then she continued, "Sweetheart, let me tell you something. It's hard when you're disabled and can't walk. After the car accident, I can't go anywhere without my guide dog."

I said nothing and let her statement settle in the air between us. There was no guide dog to be found. I felt sympathy for her pain and the fact that she now used a wheelchair to get around, but again, something wasn't quite adding up.

"Where is your dog today?" I asked innocently. Ms. Clark didn't break eye contact for a moment and acted as if she hadn't heard my question.

"I used to be able to do everything by myself. I can't even leave the house now, except to come here for my appointments," she said, tearing up.

"Hmm," I murmured, eying her freshly dyed blonde hair and beautifully manicured hands. Only a nail salon artist could have painted the intricate floral details on her acrylic nails.

At the end of our appointment, I excused myself from the room to print out Ms. Clark's visit summary. I heard a door open a few moments later and then her voice: "Excuse me, I just saw Emily Haynie."

Leila rose from her desk. "Emily will be back with you in just a minute. She's printing your visit summary. Please, go back to the room."

"Thanks, Leila," I said, stapling the printout. As I turned the corner with the visit summary in hand, I saw Ms. Clark's back as she walked, without a limp or apparent difficulty, to her room. There, she settled back into her wheelchair, sans guide dog.

"It's a miracle! She's been healed!" Leila murmured behind me, laughing to herself as she went to get my next patient from the waiting room. I stared after her incredulously before returning to Ms. Clark. *What is going on?* I wondered.

After Ms. Clark left, I learned the strange explanation for her behavior from a colleague who had seen her previously. He knew who I was referring to as soon as I said her name, a tell-tale sign that a patient is either beloved or dreaded.

Ms. Clark had been in a car accident a year ago and had sued the other driver for her resulting injuries, including back pain. She had been able to walk unassisted at her initial appointments, and both my colleague's memory and his chart notes corroborated this. At an appointment six months after the accident, however, Ms. Clark had inexplicably shown up in a wheelchair. My colleague called her out after performing a careful neurological exam and confirming she hadn't developed new weakness, but Ms. Clark steadfastly stuck to her story that she hadn't been able to walk since the accident.

I listened in amazement as he described how he ultimately zeroed in on the smoking gun. When he asked nonchalantly about how the lawsuit was going, Ms. Clark admitted that she was unhappy with the amount of money the other driver's attorney had offered as compensation. She also complained that a medical record error was causing a delay in processing her claim.

"She said I had failed to document in my original notes that she couldn't walk and was wheelchair-bound," my colleague recalled.

"No…" I breathed.

He nodded. "And here's the kicker: she asked me to make an addendum to my note saying the omission was an error so that she could send it to the attorneys. Of course, I said no. I told her that wasn't just unethical, but illegal. She got mad and said she wasn't going to see me anymore. Guess you're the lucky provider today. Thanks for taking one for the team."

"Wow" was all I could say as I absorbed the news. I'd always been a very trusting person, and I had felt genuine sympathy for Ms. Clark's back pain and reported inability to walk, even acknowledged her frustration about the attorneys dragging their feet on her claim. I felt cheated, angry that someone would lie about being disabled to get money, sympathy, attention, or whatever else. Many people really *were* disabled and didn't get any of those things. For Ms. Clark to do this and be able to live with herself made my head hurt. Yes, I screened patients for cancer and managed their cardiac risk factors and mental health. But was I really helping people? I wasn't sure anymore.

I returned to my office one afternoon after lunch to commotion coming from the waiting room.

"I don't care if he doesn't have an appointment, find one!" A woman was screaming.

As I hurried down the hall, I ran into another PA, Katie. We rounded the corner to see Bonnie, our receptionist, looking flustered, and Susie, a medical assistant, standing next to her and attempting to placate the screaming woman. Susie briefed us on the situation.

Ms. Turner had always seemed pleasant enough when I had seen her before, but today she was hysterical. She had arrived while the clinicians were out to lunch and had requested a refill of hydrocodone. Bonnie advised her that we required an appointment for all narcotic prescriptions. Ms. Turner didn't have one, and Dr. Sinclair was already double-booked for every 15-minute slot that afternoon (PAs in Texas could not prescribe schedule II-controlled substances at the time).

"Will you just ask if he can squeeze me in? It should take, like, five minutes," Ms. Turner had said impatiently.

"I'll ask him, but I want to let you know his schedule is completely full right now."

"That's fine, I'll wait."

Bonnie located Dr. Sinclair, who promptly denied the request for a same-day appointment. Ms. Turner was a long-time patient, and he reiterated the policy regularly at her follow-ups. She could put her name down on the waiting list for next week.

Ms. Turner then unleashed her rage. She swung her purse at Bonnie's head (and luckily missed), screamed an obscenity at her, and started berating her for not doing her job, even as other patients filed into the waiting room.

"Tell him I'm down to my last pill of hydrocodone, and I'll come in next week. He just needs to write me enough until then!"

But Bonnie remained firm. "I understand, but unfortunately we can't do that for this kind of controlled medicine."

Ms. Turner, embroiled in her fury, dissolved into tears and began wailing. Now Dr. Sinclair was marching toward us.

"She's lost her mind," he muttered, indicating for Katie and me to follow without slowing his pace. "Her neurologist already dismissed her for bad behavior, but I'm still responsible as her PCP." He strode through the waiting room door.

"Ms. Turner, I'm going to need you to calm down," Dr. Sinclair ordered authoritatively.

If there was anything I'd learned from dealing with angry people before that point, it was that "please calm down" or any variation thereof inevitably had the opposite effect. I braced for an explosion.

"I don't need to calm down. I need my pain meds!" Ms. Turner shrieked.

Katie and I stood by uncertainly as we stared at the black eyeliner staining her cheeks like war paint. Dr. Sinclair, however, was unmoved. He towered above Ms. Turner. I had never noticed how tall he was before that.

"This is inexcusable. We're going to have to let you go if you continue to behave inappropriately," he said in a warning tone.

"You can't do that!" Ms. Turner protested.

"Yes, we can. You're a responsible adult, and you know our policy. Everyone else here made an appointment, and you're being disrespectful by making a scene."

"Please make an exception for me," Ms. Turner whimpered. "I'm in so much pain, and I need my hydros."

Dr. Sinclair sighed, then said in a gentler tone, "I'm sorry, Ms. Turner. I'm seeing thirty patients this afternoon. Why don't you sit down for a minute, and schedule with Bonnie for my next available appointment. I suggest you apologize to her."

With that, he turned to leave. Suddenly, Ms. Turner prostrated herself in front of him and grabbed him around the ankle to keep him from going back through the door. Next thing I knew, we were all in the melee. After he wrestled his leg from her desperate grasp, Dr. Sinclair picked up the phone on Bonnie's desk and called hospital security.

Some minutes later, officers escorted Ms. Turner out. We could still hear her bawling all the way down the hall.

"Are you going to fire her?" Katie asked Dr. Sinclair breathlessly.

"I have to," he replied sadly. "She's the one who damaged the relationship with her bad behavior. She's assaulting employees. Will you both create an entry in her chart? I'll do mine after the afternoon patients. This mess has already made me late."

Katie and I nodded silently. Just as a spouse can file for divorce due to "irreconcilable differences," a clinician can determine that a relationship has become "irreparably damaged" by a patient's inappropriate behavior, ongoing noncompliance with treatment, failure to pay for services the clinician has already executed, and so forth. Inappropriate behavior may result in immediate termination because it demonstrates a patient's loss of respect or trust for the clinician. Depending on the behavior, it may also constitute criminal trespassing, assault, or deadly conduct.

In most cases, Dr. Sinclair later told me, we give patients numerous "second chances" before making the decision to cut ties. Patients have the right to feel upset, and we must remain compassionate even once we request that they correct their behavior. We took an oath to care for them, relieve their pain and suffering, and help them overcome barriers to compliance. Thus, we often continue to work with the most stubborn or demanding patients when we would have ended the relationship long ago in any other setting.

Legal consequences were a factor as well. When Dr. Sinclair terminated Ms. Turner from our practice, the letter he signed explicitly stated that we would continue to provide her with medications for the next thirty days. This gave her time to find and contact a new medical practitioner. In addition, we would help coordinate care with the emergency department, should she require it before then.

"Think of it as a 'severance package,'" Dr. Sinclair explained. "We're communicating clearly that we're not abandoning her care by offering courtesy treatment."

"Does it protect us legally?" I asked.

"It can help. Patients can always sue, so it's important to

have the documentation to back up our decisions. That's why I had you and Katie type up what happened while it was still fresh in your minds. It can be hard to remember the details over time, and then it just becomes a 'he-said-she-said' situation. We have to spell out to the patient what behavior is unacceptable and warn them that we'll terminate them if they do it again."

I silently mulled this over. It would have been nice to have had more discussions about our legal rights and responsibilities in PA school, but I suppose they didn't want to scare us away before we even started our careers.

Mr. McKnight was another one of those patients that everyone in the clinic recognized by name alone. He was Dr. Philips' patient, and I'd never personally met or seen him, but his reputation preceded him. Mr. McKnight was sixty-three years old and had chronic low back pain, depression, and anxiety. His chart also contained a special flag: *patient frequently makes false suicide threats for personal gain.*

One morning, I witnessed Mr. McKnight's showmanship firsthand. Patient appointments weren't for another fifteen minutes, and the nurse sitting next to me, Lacey, had already been there for close to an hour responding to patient messages and voicemails. She finished up on the phone with a patient and had barely said more than "good morning" to me when the phone rang shrilly again.

She glanced at the caller ID. "Look who it is. I was just thinking it's been a while since we heard from him," she remarked before picking up the receiver. "This is Lacey at Sinclair Family Practice, how may I help you?"

I heard a loud voice on the other end as I leaned over. ROBERT MCKNIGHT glowed on the display.

"Hi, Mr. McKnight," Lacey answered brightly. "I'm sorry to

hear your back's been hurting. Let me see if Dr. Philips has any cancellations. There weren't any when I last checked yesterday." She scrolled on her screen. "Okay ... uh huh, I understand ... I'm looking at her schedule right now, and she doesn't have any cancellations, but I'll send her a message so she knows what's going on. She may be able to prescribe you something."

"I need to see her NOW!" I heard Mr. McKnight's response even without the speakerphone. Lacey didn't bat an eye and remained the picture of perfect calm.

"Mr. McKnight, I'll call you back as soon as Dr. Philips gives me an answer, okay?"

"You don't understand! The pain is a 12 out of 10!"

"I recommend you go to the ER if it's that severe. They may be able to get you some relief in the meantime ... Yes, it's up to you, but we don't want you to suffer." I was always amazed by Lacey's ability to be perky in the mornings, and even more so by her remaining pleasant and accommodating as the phone rang off the hook for eight more hours. She, the schedulers, and the medical assistants were always the first to arrive in the morning when we clinicians were still trying to wake ourselves up with coffee.

Lacey put the receiver back on the hook as I stood up to see my first patient of the day.

"He hung up on me," she said, shrugging and finishing her documentation of their call. I shook my head before walking away.

"I don't know how you do it," I told her candidly.

Imagine my surprise when I returned twenty minutes later to hear Lacey on the phone with Mr. McKnight. Again. What was he calling about now?

By the time I discharged my next patient, Lacey had finally disentangled herself from the phone lines. Apparently, Mr. McKnight had regrouped after hanging up on her and decided on a different strategy. He called back ten minutes later, this time declaring, "The pain is so bad I want to kill myself." An alarming thing, of course, for anyone to hear.

Lacey, however, was well acquainted with Mr. McKnight's methods because of several similar threats he'd made in the three years that he'd been a patient at our clinic. On each occasion, he ultimately admitted that he didn't have thoughts or intentions of killing himself. He had only said these words because he couldn't handle the pain and was desperate for relief.

"So he's trying to use that as leverage? Why does Dr. Philips keep seeing him?" I cried with a flash of anger.

Lacey frowned. "She says patients in chronic pain sometimes get angry when they have trouble dealing with it. His specialists already said his back pain is stable and he doesn't need surgery, so she limited him to no more than one appointment every three months. No exceptions, even if he threatens to kill himself." She paused. "But we still have to follow hospital protocol."

She was referring to the mandatory response all employees were responsible for if a patient expressed or was otherwise at risk of suicidal thoughts, intentions, or behaviors. Suicide takes the lives of 46,000 Americans every year, so we must always take it seriously and assume the person is being truthful. Even in Mr. McKnight's case, it was always possible that one of his many seemingly empty threats was genuine. The protocol included asking about and documenting the patient's intentions, access to potential means like pills, guns, and rope, and measures to reduce the potential for an attempt. I thought of all the times I'd made calls to psychiatric treatment centers, hospital security, and relatives to make sure they were aware of a patient's risk of suicide. I'd accompanied patients to the ED or to their friends' cars so that someone always had eyes on them. I thought of the adrenaline, the anxious worry, the helplessness. How I tried to tell myself that I had done everything I could on my part.

"He doesn't know how lucky he is that I wasn't the one who answered the phone today," I said bitterly. "I have someone almost once a month who's legitimately suicidal, and it takes everything out of me to make sure they don't go through with it."

"Oh, I know," Lacey agreed earnestly. "And people like Mr. McKnight are crying wolf and wasting everybody's time, while the person who needs our help is on hold." She sighed. "You know what's sad? There are a lot more Mr. McKnights out there."

"Patients saying they're suicidal just to get what they want?"

"Yep." Lacey suddenly looked weary; she had been a nurse for many years and had long ago lost the naïveté I still possessed. My head spun with Mr. McKnight's calculatingly passive-aggressive tactics, his flagrant abuse of the health system, and Dr. Philips' benevolence. I marveled at the amount of sympathy and patience she must have, to continue to take care of someone who reserved suicidal verbiage for when he wanted an urgent appointment or an immediate response. Someone who used threats as a tactic for personal gain. Mr. McKnight demeaned the very real and overwhelming pain that consumes people who believe that taking their lives is the only solution. He sent the message that their lives were less important, that their pain was not valid. It felt wrong to keep going along with this.

Noncompliance

Although common and a familiar concept to any clinician, the "noncompliant patient" is anything but straightforward. It wasn't until I met Ms. Wilson that I first appreciated this. A 67-year-old woman from Abilene, Texas, Ms. Wilson had perfectly coiffed blonde hair and a sugary southern drawl. She always dressed impeccably, adorning her slender frame with bright sweaters and delicate jewels. She followed a Mediterranean diet, enjoyed an occasional glass of chardonnay, stuck to an enviable sleep routine, and kept her porcelain skin moisturized and well protected from the sun. As a result, she had aged like a fine wine and looked about ten years younger than she was.

A few times a year, Ms. Wilson made the three-hour drive to Dallas to see us for her hypertension, hyperlipidemia, arthritis, and seasonal allergies. There were family practices much closer to where she lived, but she had first come to us when a painful ear infection interrupted her vacation and had been a loyal patient ever since.

At her most recent appointment, I had caught a whiff of stale cigarette smoke while performing Ms. Wilson's physical exam. She also wore perfume that smelled of musk, but every now and then, there it was, that unmistakable scent. I referred to the social history in her chart: *Former smoker, cigarettes. 20 pack-years. Quit in 2006.* I knew she had quit several times throughout her life, for varying periods of time.

"Ms. Wilson, how long has it been since you quit smoking?" I asked casually as I sat back down.

"Oh, that was forever ago! Maybe ten years now," she replied.

"I thought so. Does anyone smoke at home? I'm asking because I smell some cigarette smoke right now," I said cautiously.

A look of surprise flickered across Ms. Wilson's face, and she seemed to consider pinning it on a family member for a second. Then she sighed and absentmindedly touched the emerald pendant on her necklace before looking at me again.

"I've had a few cigarettes since my mother died," she admitted.

"How many, would you say, in a day?"

"Honestly, I'm not sure ... Maybe half a pack, if that? Some days I'll only have a couple cigarettes. It's strange, but I feel like it's the only thing that I have left of her."

"Oh, Ms. Wilson, you know that's not true. You have all those pictures ... and memories!"

"I know," she replied sadly. "The smell just reminds me of her. We used to sit on her porch when it was cold out. She'd smoke a cigarette and I'd have a cup of hot cider. Sometimes it's like I can feel her there with me when I'm smoking. It calms my nerves."

I bit my lip. Now wasn't the time to launch into a lecture on why smoking was bad, but I was also responsible for encouraging patients at every visit to avoid tobacco. How could I do that compassionately and discourage something she associated so strongly with someone she loved?

I knew that Ms. Wilson had had a horrible time grieving her mother after she died the previous year. She had seen me often in those first few months because she developed a new, all-consuming anxiety. She still forced herself to go to book club, church, and lunches with her girlfriends as if everything was fine, but she could not shake the feeling of constant worry and dread that something bad was going to happen. She worried whether her children, who were all doing well in their careers and had wonderful families, had everything they wanted in life. She worried about her husband's health and her neighbor's health and the cat's health. She worried about stories she saw on the news, and she even became fearful of activities she had previously enjoyed, like driving.

At the same time, Ms. Wilson refused every last one of her family's and my recommendations for medication, therapy, or a grief support group. She worried about the possible side effects of mood medications, and what other people would think if they learned that she relied on medicine or a shrink. While some of her fears were understandable, some of them also met the definition of insanity of "doing the same thing over and over and expecting different results." Her anxiety had paralyzed her.

Maybe a month after her mother died, someone walked past Ms. Wilson at the store and smelled like cigarettes.

"It was like I forgot for a moment that she was gone, and I just bought a box at the counter on my way out," Ms. Wilson admitted.

With that first long drag, she felt some of her anxiety dissipate into the air with her breath. Nothing else had been able to give her that comfort. She began sneaking out to the alley behind her garage to smoke a cigarette here or there under the guise of tending to her garden. She was ashamed of her secret; she felt like she had let her family down because they had been so happy when she quit all those years ago.

I listened quietly, feeling a pang of dread at the thought of losing my own parents. I couldn't imagine the interminable sorrow in the absence of people who had been there all my life. Even though we lived in different cities now, I could still call them and hear their voices anytime. They still comforted and encouraged me when I had a hard day at work or felt sad or angry. Who would be there for me when they were gone?

"I can't possibly know how much you miss her," I acknowledged gently. "Tell your family and friends when you feel down or anxious. They want to listen and be there for you, just like I do."

Ms. Wilson looked away. "I just don't want to be a burden. It's been almost a year since I lost her."

"That doesn't mean you miss her any less," I said. "No one tells us how we're supposed to cope. It may help you to find new ways to remember your mother. Whatever you choose, my job is to help you stay healthy. I would love to help you quit smoking again when you're ready." I gave Ms. Wilson what I hoped was an understanding smile. "What do you think about following up a little sooner this time? Say, in a month, so we can continue our conversation?"

"Alright, then," she agreed.

I didn't see Ms. Wilson again until just before her seventieth birthday, when her husband unexpectedly died from a heart attack. By then, she had developed a feeble, helpless cough. It sounded on the one hand like she was not strong enough to cough anything up and, on the other hand, like she was drowning in her own saliva. The around-the-clock nicotine suppressed her appetite, and her already petite, thin figure had slowly shrunk, accentuating bones and wrinkles I had never noticed before.

After she nearly tipped over from a particularly intense bout of coughing, I jumped on the moment to revisit the idea of quitting.

"I've been watching, and you're using these accessory muscles because your regular breathing muscles can't keep up with moving air in and out," I told her. I gestured to my neck and collarbone. "There's air all around you, and your body shouldn't have to work so hard just to breathe. Let me help you be free of these cigarettes again. You'll feel a whole lot better."

Ms. Wilson waved the suggestion away dismissively, although she did eventually consent to a screening CT scan for lung cancer. Thankfully, it was negative. My smoking cessation counseling apparently had no impact otherwise. A few months later, Ms. Wilson fell asleep with a lit cigarette in her hand, and her house caught fire. Her son called our clinic from the hospital to tell me this. Fortunately, Ms. Wilson was alive, although she had second degree burns on her body and half of her home was gone. The doctors portended a fair prognosis, but cautioned that it would take longer for the burns to heal because she was a heavy smoker. She was up to one and a half packs per day now.

"They asked her to stop just for the time that she's in the hospital and gave her nicotine patches," Ms. Wilson's son told me. "But now she's just wearing three nicotine patches and smoking at the same time." That call drained me. *Noncompliance* used to be a simple term for a patient rejecting a clinician's medical recommendations, thereby causing or worsening his or her health conditions. Ms. Wilson was noncompliant in every sense of the word. She refused to quit harmful behaviors like smoking, which increased her risks for cancer, heart disease, and diabetes, and which worsened her hypertension. She refused medication, therapy, or healthy coping mechanisms for emotional distress, limiting her capacity to effectively control her anxiety and function better despite her grief. But Ms. Wilson's noncompliance didn't affect only her. Her family suffered the effects of her denial and addictions too. Ultimately, it was them who I felt I had let down.

My heart sank a little further when I saw the patient's name after Ms. Wilson's on my schedule that day. Ms. Ferguson was nearly the same age and had been smoking since she was eighteen years old. She had chronic obstructive pulmonary disease (COPD), gastroesophageal reflux disease (GERD), hypertension, and several other comorbidities associated with or exacerbated by smoking. Like Ms. Wilson, Ms. Ferguson was a sweet lady with a big heart who I couldn't help but have a soft spot for.

"How have you been?" I asked her with a sunny smile, even though I didn't feel particularly sunny.

"Good, good. I'm just here for refills," Ms. Ferguson responded.

"Alright, let's make sure I have everything up to date here. You're still taking 10 mg of amlodipine for your blood pressure?"

"Yes."

"And your albuterol inhaler, the as-needed one, how often are you using it for your breathing?"

Ms. Ferguson let out a small squeal and grinned. "I was waiting for you to ask me that! I use it just here and there now. I quit smoking two months ago."

"You quit?! That's great news!" I was now the one grinning from ear to ear, at once surprised and delighted. After I went through the remainder of her medication list, Ms. Ferguson recounted the pivotal event that finally tipped the scales and helped her quit her years-long habit. Tears welled up in her eyes as she told me the story.

"My grandbaby came and sat on my lap while I was smoking. She said, 'Gramma, I wish you would stop. I don't want you to die.' And that was it. I threw away the pack of cigarettes I had on me, and I haven't smoked one since."

"This is huge," I said, reaching for her hand. "Your family asks you to stop all the time, but she really moved you."

Ms. Ferguson nodded through tears. "She's incredible. I told her, 'Gramma doesn't want to die, either.' I want to be around to watch my grandbaby grow up." Ms. Ferguson showed me a photo of the adorable little girl on her cell phone. She had no formal education or medical training. Nevertheless, she had achieved what all the adults in Ms. Ferguson's life, myself included, had not.

When I saw Ms. Ferguson six months and then a year later, she remained smoke-free and reported she did not miss it one bit. She breathed better and required fewer inhalers, and her hypertension and obesity had improved as she gradually tolerated more activity. It lifted my spirits to hear about each progressive success and the meaning it added to her life. Meanwhile, Ms. Wilson was still smoking like a chimney and had been diagnosed with macular degeneration. She would likely go blind within the next ten years, maybe even five because smoking added fuel to the fire.

I wished I could make Ms. Ferguson a spokesperson for all the Ms. Wilsons out there who weren't ready to quit. She reminded me why I kept enduring when patients resisted change, and why we search tirelessly for the one reason that matters enough to move the needle. If I gave up, my patients would, too. Ms. Ferguson's story also served as a warning. In the practice of medicine, the lows could be very low. It was easy to carry the feeling of futility from one patient's appointment into the next. But every patient deserved a full tank from me. I had to counteract hopelessness and frustration with the joy of healing those who sought my help. I had to celebrate the triumphs; otherwise, I would almost certainly perish.

POSSIBLE SIDE EFFECT: MURDER

R*IIIIIING.* My eyes roved around the walls of an unfamiliar room as they echoed sound back to me from all directions at once. I stared, mesmerized, at their shimmering, liquid appearance. Even though I had no clue where I was, I knew the ringing phone and the waiting patients were for me. I was asleep, but they wouldn't allow me to rest, even in my dreams.

RIIIIIING. I groaned and rolled over in bed as consciousness slowly crept in. My cell phone blared next to my head on the nightstand, its bright screen glowing with ON CALL PAGE. The only thing worse than dreaming about being paged was waking up to find out it wasn't a dream. It was 4:07 a.m., and I had just barely fallen back asleep after a page at 2:30 a.m. A father had asked if he should take his 16-year-old daughter to the ED because she had started with a fever two hours ago. Her highest temperature was 99.8°F, she had no other symptoms, and she was otherwise healthy. I reassured him that there was nothing to warrant an emergency, and he agreed to bring her in when our clinic opened at 8:00 a.m. if he felt like she needed medical attention or testing. The father then asked what she could take for the fever, as if in sixteen years he had never had to treat either his child or himself for this mysterious ailment. I had politely advised a dose of Tylenol.

I flung my arm out and brought the demanding inanimate object to my ear, wondering if this page was him calling again.

"Hello?" I mumbled sleepily.

"This is the answering service with a page for Emily Haynie," a chipper voice responded on the other end.

"Speaking."

"I have your patient, Karen Bell, date of birth 05/22/77, calling about a problem with her medication. Can I put you through?"

"Just a minute." I shivered as I emerged from my beloved pillowy comforter and lowered my bare feet onto the cold hardwood floor. My dislike of being cold was second only to my dislike of being tired; right now, both were accosting me at once. I reached for my laptop on the dresser and robotically logged into the EMR. After I typed in the DOB the page operator gave me, Ms. Bell's photo appeared on the screen. I recognized her face; she was a nice lady who saw me some months back for a well woman exam.

"Okay, you can put her through," I said to the operator, scanning Ms. Bell's medication list. "Hi, Ms. Bell, it's Emily Haynie, the PA. Can you tell me what's going on?"

No one spoke. Instead, I heard breathing, fast and deep like that of the patients I'd seen in the ED with diabetic ketoacidosis (DKA). Kussmaul breathing, sometimes called "air hunger" because of the exaggerated effort and sound of someone starved for air, is actually an uncontrollable kind of hyperventilation to expel the body's excess acid. Watching it was like witnessing life drift out of a human being. Children in DKA, especially, seemed so weak and helpless that I felt their desperation.

"Ms. Bell, can you hear me?" I called out nervously.

The breathing finally paused, followed by a horrifying response. "I think my medication made me kill someone."

"What—where are you?" Suddenly I was wide awake.

"I'm in my house. I . . . woke up in my car and there was blood all over my head. I don't know what to do."

"Did you call 911?"

"No, I was too scared. My husband said to call you first."

"Why?" I cried. "I need you to call 911. Are you still bleeding? Did someone hurt you? Are you still with them?" I was talking so fast in my shock that Ms. Bell didn't even have a chance to respond. I hardly knew what I was saying myself.

"I'm not bleeding anymore, and I don't know where the person is," Ms. Bell eventually interjected into my babbling. "I went to bed last night, took my sleeping pill, and then I woke up in my car. I can't remember anything." She confirmed the name and dose of her sleep medication since I didn't see it in her chart. She told me her psychiatrist had prescribed it after a warning that, rarely, people did weird stuff in their sleep after taking it. Ms. Bell had never sleepwalked, so her risk of these side effects was low.

"I've taken it several times, and nothing's ever happened," she insisted. "Last night, the medicine didn't work, so I took a second pill."

"How long did it take you to fall asleep?"

"I don't know. I still can't remember anything after that. My Ring camera shows me backing up into the street in the middle of the night and hitting someone." I inhaled sharply.

"Did they get out of the car?"

"They weren't driving . . . they were walking. You can see them go down." I involuntarily covered my mouth with my hand and listened with increasing horror as she continued. "It looks like I just sat in the same spot and then at some point, I drove back into the garage and stayed there for like an hour before I got out."

"And the person . . ."

"There wasn't anyone in the street when my husband and I checked, but my back bumper is messed up, and I think the blood on my face is from hitting my head on the steering wheel. I would never hurt anyone; that's not me." Ms. Bell's voice shook, like she was trying to convince herself that she was speaking the truth. *She didn't call 911 after she watched the Ring video?* This was not the kind of urgent call the after-hours service was meant for. I was suddenly reminded of a conversation I'd had with another patient, Ms. Wright, about a possible side effect on her Wellbutrin prescription information sheet.

"Murder. Forceful actions, fury, anxiety, and anger," Ms. Wright had read aloud to me as I tried to maintain a serious expression. I didn't want to appear to downplay her concerns. I had prescribed Wellbutrin for Ms. Wright because it was an FDA-approved medicine for smoking cessation, but it also treated depression and ADHD. I explained to Ms. Wright that someone who took Wellbutrin reported thoughts of murder, or worst-case scenario, they killed someone. But just because that person believed his or her thoughts and the medicine were related did not prove that they were, or that Wellbutrin caused them. It was always possible that people taking Wellbutrin for depression were misdiagnosed or had more than one mental health condition. Homicidal thoughts were more common with schizophrenia and personality disorders, but they could happen with depression and bipolar disorder, too. I had reassured Ms. Wright that she wasn't going to murder anyone, and we had both laughed about it after the fact.

Now, it felt like my tongue was so fat it was filling up my mouth. I knew what I wanted to say, but it was hard to get the words out.

"Ms. Bell, from what you've told me, I need to call the police. We have to find out if you hurt or killed someone, even if it was an accident."

"I'm so scared," she said in a pleading voice.

"I know, but we have to tell them. You may need to go to the hospital, too, to get examined."

Ms. Bell didn't say anything, but I could hear her sniffling. After she confirmed her address and her husband promised they'd stay put, I documented our conversation and recounted it for the police. They told me they'd be in touch. By now, it was 5:00 a.m., and there was no way I was going back to sleep. My thoughts swirled as I got ready and left for work. I'd never been the first one there before.

Later that week, Ms. Bell sobbed with relief as she told me that she had not killed anyone and wasn't going to jail. She had backed her car into a runner, who didn't hear her coming because he was wearing noise-cancelling headphones and had his back to her. Although he had fractured his pelvis, the runner was alive and expected to make a full recovery because he was young and healthy. Ms. Bell wasn't taking any chances, though; she had already flushed the rest of her sleeping pills down the toilet.

HEARTBREAK

As my experience and confidence grew, I realized that my purpose as a PA was not to be the all-knowing professional in the white coat. It was not to show people the "right" way to be healthy. Rather, it was to encourage them to take an active part in their healthcare. The *way* I went about this was determined, I believe, by what Dr. Sinclair had described as "figuring out a patient's personality." My personal effectiveness as a clinician depended on my ability to interpret my patients' behaviors and personal values, and to adapt my role accordingly. Detective, therapist, designer, advocate, teacher... I used my medical knowledge to provide accurate information about risks and benefits so that patients could make informed decisions. In doing so, I gradually became less paternalistic and more of a partner in their care. However, there were always conditions I had never encountered, life scenarios I had never experienced.

In 2000, an entertaining reality TV show called *Cheaters* aired on The CW Plus. The show followed a different person each week who suspected that a significant other was cheating. A wife would burst out of a decoy vehicle, catch her unfaithful husband in the act like a deer in the headlights, and publicly out him with next-level rage. It was satisfying to see the camera crew swarm in as the wife screamed and threw things at her husband; they'd heckle both the husband and the other woman, invariably inciting an even bigger brawl.

It was much tougher to see the effects of infidelity on

my patients, people I cared about. A 35-year-old woman named Ms. Beeman made an appointment with me one day complaining of stroke-like symptoms. The nurse alerted me immediately; a stroke is a medical emergency because it can result in permanent damage to the brain. Treatment, if safe to administer, must be given within a few hours of the symptoms starting, so time is of the essence. Ms. Beeman reassured us that she'd already been to the ED and that the symptoms had actually happened several months ago, so I allowed her to come in and give me the full story.

While delivering a presentation at work, Ms. Beeman had suddenly felt numbness and tingling on the left side of her face. Her tongue felt like it weighed ten pounds. She continued to speak, but when her words sounded funny, her coworkers rushed her to the ED. Fortunately, her brain scans were normal, and her symptoms had already started improving within a few hours. The doctors also ruled out a transient ischemic attack (TIA), in which symptoms resolve within 24 hours, and which can precede a permanent stroke. Ms. Beeman was a healthy young woman without any personal or family risk factors, so the ED team concluded that sleep deprivation, dehydration, and stress about the presentation were to blame. She saw a neurologist, too, who agreed with the diagnosis.

Ms. Beeman admitted that she had a different explanation, one that she had not shared with anyone else until now because it was too painful. The night before the presentation, she had found out that her husband of almost ten years was cheating on her. Worse, he wanted *her* to move out of the house they shared because he planned to have the other woman move in! She didn't sleep at all that night and cried her eyes out instead ("so at least the part about sleep deprivation and dehydration were probably accurate," she told me). She floundered her way through an important presentation, even though she knew the information backwards and forwards.

After the ED, Ms. Beeman had lived in an extended stay hotel temporarily so she could figure out what to do. When she returned home to get some different clothes for work, she saw the other woman's clothes hanging in the bedroom closet—her closet—and a photo of her husband and his side chick on the nightstand. It was like she had never existed. They hadn't even filed for divorce yet! She thought she was going to throw up and have a stroke for real this time. She left without grabbing a single thing and vowed never to step foot in that house again. And then she scheduled this appointment with me.

I conveyed my shock and sympathy at such a crushing betrayal. I didn't have a solution to Ms. Beeman's emotional pain and its physical manifestations, but I reassured her that she—not her husband, and certainly not his mistress—was my patient, so I would do everything in my ability to care for her well-being. I connected her with a trusted psychiatrist, who prescribed medication, intensive therapy, and direct involvement from her friends and family. Gradually, I witnessed her transformation into a woman who was able to find love again.

Ms. Beeman's ex-husband, meanwhile, met a fate far worse than that in any episodes of *Cheaters*. His mistress divorced him after a few years and took full custody of their two children. There were rumors of domestic violence, and his reputation in their small town suffered until the day came when he took his own life. Despite the years of anger, pain, and loneliness her ex had caused her, Ms. Beeman's heart broke for him anew. Through her, I saw that people can grieve the loss of relationships, even when someone deeply wrongs or hurts us. We go through the same stages of denial, anger, bargaining, depression, and, in the best-case scenario, acceptance. Love is often inseparable from pain and suffering.

While other stories of cheating were less sensational,

patients nevertheless came to me in a similar state of shock. One morning, a 19-year-old man who had been my patient for several years checked in at the front desk for a "private consultation." Usually friendly and relaxed, today he was visibly nervous and fidgeted on the exam table.

"What can I help you with today?" I asked.

"My girlfriend told me yesterday that she cheated on me," he responded morosely.

"Oh no, Nate, I'm so sorry. You two have been together a long time."

"Yeah, two years. She swears it was just one time but… I just don't know how she could do this to me." He looked like he was about to cry.

"This is a lot for you to deal with. I can't imagine what you're feeling, but just let yourself feel it; don't hold it in. I'm here for *you*."

"She got an STD from him," Nate blurted out, his face reddening. "She said she took medicine for it, and it's gone. But now I have this watery stuff coming out of my…" He motioned towards his lap and exhaled forcefully. "My dick. I don't know what the medical term is."

It took every ounce of professionalism to keep a straight face and look Nate in the eyes. He was clearly in distress, as any normal person would be, after this double whammy from his girlfriend.

"It's penis," I said gently. "I'm going to treat you and do some testing to make sure you didn't get anything else. Is that okay with you?"

As if contemplating the origins of the universe, he nodded slowly, his thoughts far, far away. Finally, he said, "Right, my penis. That makes sense. Yeah, I'm fine with doing some tests."

I'm happy to say that Nate's condition was easily cured. While his heartbreak took much longer to heal, eventually it did, too. Last year, he introduced me to his fiancée, and I had the chance to wish them a wonderful life together. Life is often unkind, but I learned that our capacity to love is amazing and can prevail even in the most unlikely circumstances.

DIEGO GOES TO THE DOCTOR

Once, I walked into an exam room and thought for several horrifying minutes that the patient was dead. Mr. Roberts, a 60-year-old man, had been waiting alone in the room for about half an hour. I was running behind because my last patient showed up late, and no one had checked on Mr. Roberts in the meantime. He sat slumped over in a chair, motionless.

"Mr. Roberts?"

He didn't stir. I moved closer, my heartbeat quickening.

"Mr. Roberts?" I repeated, louder this time as I gently shook his shoulder. Suddenly, he grunted and let out a loud snore. I smelled liquor on his breath and sighed. At least he wasn't dead.

After a few more moments, Mr. Roberts stretched, blinked, and looked around the room like he couldn't remember how he got there. His eyes were red and glazed, and dry spittle collected at the corner of his mouth.

"Hi, Mr. Roberts. You tired today?" *And by that, I mean, are you drunk?*

"Yeah, sorry about that. I didn't get much sleep last night; me and my ex been at it again."

"What happened?" I asked as I checked his pupils. They were dilated and slow to respond to bright light.

"Well, you know we've been separated."

"Yes, I remember."

"And I was sober for four months. I was doing real good."

"I'm happy to hear that. It was hard for you to be sober around her."

Mr. Roberts rubbed his temples. "Yeah, she's a real piece of work. She doesn't want to be with me anymore, but she still gets jealous if she even hears that I'm talking to someone. It could be the lady who delivers the mail, or the cashier at the grocery store. Doesn't make any difference to that crazy woman."

Even though I had never met her, I felt like I was well acquainted with Mr. Roberts' ex-wife from all the stories he had told me. For one, she could drink him under the table. She was a tiny 5'1" woman whose volatile temper intensified with each incremental increase in blood alcohol content. I remembered Mr. Roberts telling me that, once, when he didn't answer his phone because he didn't feel it vibrate in his coat pocket, she logged onto his laptop, found his location by searching for the phone, called once more (it went to voicemail again), and drove to the bar where he was. She jumped to the conclusion that Mr. Roberts was cheating on her, when he was in fact there with a close guy friend, blowing off steam after work. Without going inside to confirm, his wife walked over to his car, slashed the tires, and smashed the windshield in with a landscaping brick from their front yard. Security cameras captured the footage, and she got a misdemeanor charge, but it was Mr. Roberts who had to pay for the repairs.

This time, Mr. Roberts told me, he had come home to find his house ransacked. He thought someone had robbed him. Drawers and cabinets were open and rifled through; broken picture frames, electronics, and tchotchkes littered the floor; and the money that he hid in a locked file cabinet was gone. Only when he checked the home security system video did he see the woman who used to be the love of his life crashing through the house like a steer in the Running of the Bulls. Mr. Roberts wanted to kick himself for being so stupid; she didn't have a key anymore, but she still knew the code to disarm the security system. And of course, she knew where he hid the money. He changed all the codes and locks that night.

"That's smart," I remarked.

He shook his head. "She didn't like that. Yesterday, I was backing out of the driveway and her car was right there, blocking me in so I couldn't leave. She had driven right over the grass, and there were tire tracks and mud everywhere. It looked like a tornado came through."

One of their many terrible fights followed. His ex looked like shit and was so drunk she could barely stand, he said. When she finally left, she screeched out of the driveway and took off with his mailbox on the hood of her car. Mr. Roberts was so furious and distracted that he didn't even realize what he was doing: muscle memory took him straight to the liquor store. As much as he hated to admit it, that first drink was like the nectar of the gods after the drought of sobriety and the insanity of his ex.

"Did you drink anything today?" I asked.

"Well… yeah, I had a little."

"How much is a little?"

"A six-pack of Tall Boys." He hesitated, then sheepishly added, "And a handle of vodka. I figured if I finished it off, there wouldn't be any more alcohol in the house."

I glanced down at my watch. "It's only 10:00 a.m., Mr. Roberts. Did you drive yourself here?"

"Probably shouldn't have done that, huh."

Our conversation was somehow turning into the real-life version of a TikTok video my friend had showed me called "The Doctor Visit," which features two puppets. The doctor asks the patient routine questions about tobacco, alcohol, and drug use to obtain an adequate social history. The latter's first instinct is to deny everything, and he hesitantly reveals a little bit of the truth only after continued prodding and rephrasing of supposedly yes or no questions:

Doctor: Diego, nice to see you again.
Patient: Hello, doctor.
Doctor: You here for your annual checkup?
Diego: Yes.
Doctor: Good, good. Before we get started, how's everything been?
Diego: Eh, you know… still married, so…
Doctor: You know what they say: "the secret to a happy marriage remains a secret."
Diego: Oh… that, that doesn't help me at all.
Doctor: Do you smoke?
Diego: No.
Doctor: You sure?
Diego: No.
Doctor: You're not sure.
Diego: I mean, I occasionally have a cigarette or… a joint… or crack.
Doctor: It's a yes or no answer, Diego.
Diego: Okay, yes.
Doctor: Do you drink?
Diego: No.
Doctor: Are you sure?
Diego: I mean, like casually, at a party or a wedding or something like that. (pauses) Or at my house, alone… every night.
Doctor: What do you drink?
Diego: Just like, a glass of wine with dinner.
Doctor: Okay, that's healthy.
Diego: And then a shot of tequila.
Doctor: Okay…

Diego: And then another shot.
Doctor: Um—
Diego: And a few more. And then some more. And then I usually pass out. And I wake up, and I take a few more.
Doctor: So... the answer is yes. Do you do any drugs?
Diego: No.
Doctor: Are you sure.
Diego: I mean, occasionally I'll smoke a little weed here and there. I'll do a little blow at a party, some shrooms... nothing crazy.
Doctor: Yes, or no?
Diego: Yes, I take drugs.
Doctor: Any prescription pills or over the counter medicine?
Diego: No.
Doctor: You sure?
Diego: I mean, I take Advil and Tylenol, stuff like that.
Doctor: How often?
Diego: Um, every time my wife talks to me.
Doctor: Why?
Diego: Because I know it's going to give me a headache.
Doctor: So... the answer is yes.
Diego: Yes.

I couldn't stop laughing the first time I watched this video all the way through. The puppets' unchanging expressions coupled with their deadpan conversation somehow seemed even more spot-on than if the video had featured live actors. I'd now been in the doctor's position many times and had stopped taking patients' social history answers at face value, other than the ones about their occupations. I had stopped taking patients' social history answers at face value. I remember the first time I had thought that I needed to be more specific when asking about substance use. A young man had come in complaining of poor sleep and daytime sleepiness, and although sleep apnea was first on my differential, I suspected substances might be a major contributor.

"Do you use any illegal drugs?" I asked him, like I had many times since I learned it in PA school.

"No," he responded, despite the unmistakable smell of marijuana on him.

I paused.

"Do you smoke weed?"

"Yeah, sometimes," he answered casually with a shrug.

"When's the last time you smoked?"

"I had some last weekend when I was in California."

"Well, it's still illegal in Texas, don't forget," I responded, looking him dead in the eye and feeling like a D.A.R.E. instructor. He nodded, unconcerned.

"Yeah, I know. I only do it when I'm in California or Colorado."

I'm sure you do, I thought, making a mental note to explicitly ask patients in the future about their exposure to common illicit drugs, one by one. Other patients would offer similar explanations of smoking weed only in California or Colorado, but I was wiser now. I learned to ask different questions about alcohol use, too: "How many days a week do you usually have a drink? What's your drink of choice?"

Presently, I finished my exam of Mr. Roberts and told him, "I'd like to order some bloodwork to see how everything looks."

"Sure," he replied.

"Then let's get you back on the wagon. I don't want you to die or kill someone because you were drinking and driving. Plus, we're not going to let her win; you're stronger than that."

He sighed. "I'm glad there's someone out here who cares about me. That woman just messes with my head. I gotta get right."

I turned to the computer to order the tests and racked my brain for a good plan forward. Mr. Roberts lived alone, and his children weren't nearby or involved in his care. I took it as a good sign that, even though he had relapsed, he had showed up in our office the very next day and expressed a desire to get sober again.

Suddenly, Mr. Roberts interrupted my thoughts. "Uh, Emily? I gotta be honest… I've been doing some cocaine, too."

SELF-HARM VIA MARINE LIFE

Most common International Classification of Diseases, tenth edition (ICD-10) codes in primary care, which clinicians select during an appointment when we make a diagnosis:

I10	Primary (Essential) hypertension
J45	Asthma
E11.9	Type 2 Diabetes Mellitus
Z91.1	Patient's noncompliance with medical treatment and regimen

A sampling of my favorite ICD-10 codes, which I became aware of after initially searching for a diagnosis of "injury," and which, fortunately, I have not had many opportunities to use:

Y93.E2	Injury due to activity-laundry
V91.07XD	Burn due to water skis on fire
W56.01	Bitten by dolphin
W61.92	Struck by other birds
W59.11XA	Struck by a turtle
W22.02	Walked into lamppost
V9540Xa	Unspecified spacecraft accident injuring occupant
V9733XA	Sucked into jet engine
T63.612	Toxic effect of contact with Portuguese Man-o-war, intentional self-harm

I have so. Many. Questions.

FOR THE LIVING

Eventually, I was tasked with communicating a new diagnosis of cancer to a patient. I knew that it would happen if I worked in medicine long enough, but that was no comfort when the moment came. A 70-year-old patient who was usually active and energetic had told me she felt exhausted and had lost a significant amount of weight without trying. In the last few weeks, she had also developed new low back pain and difficulty walking. I ordered a spine x-ray, which showed abnormal changes in the bones; and blood tests, which showed high levels of inflammatory markers that were equally concerning. With a leaden feeling in the pit of my stomach, I called the patient and asked her to come in so we could go over the results together.

"I'm not coming back in," she said. "I was there two days ago. Just tell me what they are over the phone."

"Ms. Martin, it's really important for us to talk about these in person," I pleaded. "I want to properly explain them to you and answer any questions you have."

"It's cancer, isn't it? Just tell me yes or no, Emily."

I fell silent, the words on the tip of my tongue. I was terrified, and my skin prickled like I was going to break out into a cold sweat.

"The test results suggest cancer, but we need more information," I finally said. Now her end went silent. Unable to stand it after a few moments, I added, "I don't think it's right to tell you over the phone like this. I'm sorry." I felt like the world's worst human being.

Ms. Martin sighed, sounding slightly annoyed that I hadn't been forthcoming with my answer. "Well, what do we do next?"

"I want you to see a specialist. I can help schedule that for you. Also, I want to get a stat MRI of your spine to get a more detailed look at what we saw on the x-ray."

"Okay, just tell me where to go."

I made several calls, and after I confirmed the details of both the MRI and oncology appointments with Ms. Martin, I hung up the phone and went straight to Dr. Sinclair. I could still barely find my words as I described the exchange with Ms. Martin in faltering sentences. Everything about it felt so wrong. *Why had I given in and told her so inhumanely, over the phone? Delivering bad news was an inevitable part of my job description, so why had school not prepared me for it?*

Dr. Sinclair sat quietly next to me and placed his hand on my shoulder. He assured me that these conversations were never easy, no matter how many times we had conducted them. He had been practicing for forty years and still hesitated, knowing that, regardless of the words he chose, the patient's life would change forever, separated into Before Cancer and After Cancer. Over time, there were a few phrases that he had decided he preferred for these serious conversations, but did any of them ever feel like the right ones? No.

When Ms. Martin returned for her follow-up appointment, Dr. Sinclair graciously accompanied me. Ms. Martin appeared very calm—much calmer than I would be if I had found out *I* had cancer—and thanked me for trying to deliver bad news compassionately. *Thanked me!* For uttering the word that no one ever wants to hear. Breast cancer that metastasized to the spine was the cause of her new back pain and weakness, the oncologist had said. While Ms. Martin had usually gotten mammograms annually, as recommended, she had skipped the last two years due to various unforeseen circumstances. She had figured she was about to be too old to need mammograms anymore, anyway. Dr. Sinclair demonstrated how to ask empathetically about how she was taking in her cancer diagnosis and what she needed from us at the present time. He expressed that both he and I would always be available for support, both inside and outside of the clinic. I waved and felt like slightly less of an awful human being as Ms. Martin checked out at the front desk.

About six months later, Dr. Sinclair told me that Ms. Martin had died. I was devastated. Death had come so quickly on the heels of my first experience delivering such terrible news. I think, deep down, I had known from the start that she would die: the breast cancer was metastatic, and therefore incurable. But I was human, so I still held out hope for a miracle.

It was Ms. Martin's husband who ultimately allowed me to feel some peace. He had been by her side when she passed, lovingly holding her hand as they laughed about a funny memory together. She had told him that she wasn't afraid to die.

"She said, 'God has been good to me; He gave me the love of my life.' She's been coming to this clinic for fifty years, and she had a wonderful quality of life because you guys took such good care of her." He managed a pained, sad smile, while I blinked hard to hold back the warmth in my eyes that meant tears weren't far behind.

"It's natural to try to stall death for as long as possible," Mr. Martin continued, as if reading my mind. "But your living patients are the ones who need you. Help them have a good quality of life so they will be less afraid when it comes."

"I'll try," I croaked, the floodgates just seconds from opening. I didn't know if I was capable of this. I was still terrified of death and how it could happen as insidiously as fatigue and a missed mammogram.

"Thank you for giving me all these years with her," Mr. Martin said.

To my surprise, he hugged me. Even more surprising, I managed not to cry.

A 40-year-old woman, Ms. Ortiz, came in for a sore throat that had lasted for three weeks. She went to an urgent care clinic initially, where she tested positive for strep throat and received a prescription for amoxicillin. When her symptoms failed to get better, she went to another doctor's office, again received the same diagnosis, and left with a prescription for clindamycin. Both antibiotics are effective treatments for group A streptococcus, the bacteria that causes strep throat, and Ms. Ortiz showed me the empty prescription bottles.

"I took everything exactly like they told me to, but it doesn't feel any better," she said hoarsely.

"We may have to do some additional tests. Let me take a look at your throat first."

When I shined my penlight at the back of her throat, it was red, swollen, and certainly looked like many cases of strep throat I had seen over the years. But when I made Ms. Ortiz say "ahh" and stick out her tongue, I saw a large, abnormal round ball on the right side of her throat. There was no similar structure on the left side, and both of her tonsils had been removed when she was a child.

"I think the reason your sore throat isn't getting better is that we're not dealing with a simple infection," I said carefully, sitting down next to her. "There is a mass behind your tongue." Ms. Ortiz shook her head but did not look shocked or scared—just frustrated.

"Can you just test me again for strep or get the doctor to take a look?"

I willingly obliged and fetched Dr. Sinclair, who shone his penlight and arrived at the same conclusion that I had. Realization started creeping across Ms. Ortiz's face.

"Are you telling me I have cancer?" she asked Dr. Sinclair. He nodded solemnly.

"Most likely, yes, it is cancer. We need to have you see a specialist as quickly as possible for treatment. You may need surgery to remove it."

As he exchanged glances with me, I remembered Ms. Martin, and how the three of us had sat together just like this as she tried to come to terms with her life-changing diagnosis. The last time I had seen her alive. I thought of my promise to Ms. Martin's husband, to care for the living and give them a good quality of life.

"We're going to take care of you," I presently said in a calm voice to the woman in front of me. I doubt she heard me through her shock.

A year later, Dr. Sinclair asked if I could join him in an exam room for a moment. I walked in and there she was, the woman with the persistent sore throat, although I almost didn't recognize her because she was much thinner. Ms. Ortiz had been treated for oropharyngeal squamous cell carcinoma and was currently in remission.

"I remember you—you're the one who found the cancer," Ms. Ortiz said, looking me dead in the eye.

"Yes, that was me." I felt like I should say sorry.

"That seems like such a long time ago," she said with a sigh.

"How are you feeling?"

"Grateful for every day that I still open my eyes and see the sun. Let me tell you, there's nothing like finding out you have cancer to get your priorities straight. I used to only be about work and never knew how to slow down and take care of myself. I didn't feel like I was doing anything right, at my job or as a mother." Ms. Ortiz and her family had moved three-

and-a-half hours away to Lake Travis, where she reacquainted herself with fresh air and sunshine. She worked a couple days a week now and spent the rest with her children. She believed that her new appreciation for life was in large part responsible for her recovery.

"I'm happy to hear that," I said, smiling. Ms. Ortiz looked at me gravely.

"It's horrible that I had to get sick to realize that wasn't a way to live. Let me give you some advice, Emily. Work to live, don't live to work. And be very thankful for every day that you get on this earth."

"Absolutely," I agreed with conviction. In fact, I did count myself lucky: I had a rewarding career as a PA and still had personal time for the things I valued. I'd made the right choice.

PART III
THE WONDER YEARS

THE SPARK

It was around the time I had been a PA for five years that I first had the idea for this book. I was in an appointment with a young man named Brian, typing up the history I'd obtained so far:

Brian Sanders
16yo M
Chief Complaint: Messed up right knee after MVA
Generalized RT knee swelling on/off x 2 mo. Initial pain and bruising resolved. Buckling sensation, stiffness after prolonged inactivity. Normal weight-bearing and range of motion. Ice, rest, ibuprofen all helpful; no treatment currently. No similar symptoms in the past.

My fingers paused on the keys, and I turned to Brian.

"You hurt your knee in a car accident, right? Were you driving, or was someone else driving?" An MVA is a motor vehicle accident.

"It wasn't a car accident. I fell," Brian said flatly. I leaned back on my stool and nodded apologetically.

"Oh, sorry. That's just what the appointment scheduler put in. Tell me how your hurt your knee, then."

Brian tossed the shaggy brown hair with bleached tips out of his eyes. Glumly, he recalled how his car had been stolen just two weeks after his parents had bought him a Suburban for his sixteenth birthday. He had left it running in the driveway while he went inside for "less than a minute" to grab his stuff for basketball practice. When he returned, he had watched in horror as two strangers jumped into his brand-new car and slammed the doors shut. Racing back into the house, Brian yelled frantically to his brother, Jeff, that he'd been carjacked.

In their excitement, neither brother thought to get into Jeff's car in the garage. Instead, they sprinted after the Suburban on foot as the thieves tried to back down the steep driveway while Brian, shouting into his phone, described his car and license plate number to the police. Just as the Suburban screeched out of the cul-de-sac and onto the main road, Brian managed to bust it on the concrete. He landed straight down on his right knee, and his cell phone flew out of his hands into the intersection. Before he could get to his feet to retrieve it, a passing car ran it over and smashed it to smithereens.

My eyes widened. I hadn't expected all this from a chief complaint of MVA.

"Did the cops ever find them?" I asked, stunned.

Brian shook his head. "No. But they found my car after a few hours. It was totaled in a ditch."

"Wow, I'm so sorry, Brian. I'm just glad they didn't shoot you or your brother. They could have had a gun."

Brian ignored me as if that was the least of his concerns. "My parents were so mad," he continued. "They were already fighting because my mom wanted me to drive my sister's old car, but my dad convinced her to get me a new one. I told Jeff he couldn't tell them I left the car running. We just said the Suburban was parked in front of the house, and they broke in and stole it."

When Brian's parents tried to file a claim with the car insurance company, things just kept getting worse. The thieves had apparently used the Suburban in a bank robbery and, after they crashed it in the ditch, they drove off in another stolen getaway car. The insurance company declined compensation while there was an ongoing criminal investigation, and Brian's mom refused to get him another car. Brian wasn't going to be caught dead driving around in his sister's "lame Volkswagen Beetle," so now he had to suck up to Jeff anytime he wanted to go somewhere.

"I hope they get that sorted out soon," I said sympathetically. I thought fondly of my first car, a used Saturn with manual windows, a cassette tape player, and a Tort Reform bumper sticker from the previous owner. It was a piece of crap, but I felt like a million bucks as I cruised around St. Louis in it as a teenager.

I turned back to the medical exam. "The x-ray of your knee was normal, but from my exam, I think you've at least partially torn your meniscus. It's a piece of cartilage between the bones that make up your knee joint."

"Oh."

"I'm going to order an MRI so we can see if that's the issue," I continued. "We can't see the meniscus on x-rays, only bones. Will you ask your mom if that's okay? MRIs can be expensive."

Brian shrugged. "She said to get whatever you think I need. She's sending everything to the insurance. They'll pay for medical bills since I messed up my knee during the robbery."

"Okay. I'll document everything you've told me so that your mom can give it to them," I assured him.

Brian suddenly looked anxious. "Wait, can she see everything you write? She still doesn't know it was my fault. Please don't tell my mom." I hid a smile. After everything that had happened, *that* was what he was worried about?

I explained that Brian was legally considered a minor since he was younger than eighteen years old, had never been married, and lived with his parents. Therefore, they must provide consent for his healthcare treatments. How involved his parents were and how much they knew depended on my clinical judgment, however. I would not tell his mom about him leaving the car running since it wasn't relevant to his knee pain treatment, but she was legally authorized to request a copy of his progress notes at any time. There was always the possibility, too, that she would find out from the insurance company, since they don't provide payment without medical records that are directly related to the injury or proof of treatment. I could not falsify or omit relevant information, especially regarding the circumstances of the incident since his case was involved in a criminal investigation.

Brian's story was the spark. I would write a book that could be adapted into a medical TV comedy based on hilarious stories and sometimes downright ludicrous encounters my colleagues and I regularly experienced with patients. An episode about MVAs would showcase Brian's story of his sweet-sixteen-present-turned-bank-heist-getaway-car. For added viewer excitement, my version would feature a high-speed police chase complete with squad cars and helicopters, like those on the show *Cops*. The Suburban would ultimately crash through someone's living room window, causing glass to scatter everywhere like a shower of diamonds, followed by a house fire of epic proportions.

My future show was tentatively titled *Family Practice: Truth Is Stranger Than Fiction*. It would star Lucy Liu as me because (a) she was an unbelievably talented actor who could nail my extra personality and inner rumination with equal perfection (this belief was later confirmed when I saw her as Simone in *Why Women Kill*); and (b) what Asian wouldn't want the strong, independent, imaginative, and stunningly gorgeous Lucy Liu to portray her?

The other patient feaured in the MVA episode would be Malcolm, a high school senior I'd taken care of who once again proved that this chief complaint, while common, was anything but ordinary.

Malcolm Petrovsky
18yo M
Chief Complaint: Checkup after MVA and possible injection

Malcolm had given me pause when he told me the reason he wanted someone to check him out in the clinic. He was running late for tennis practice the day before and had been speeding when he lost control of his car at 60 miles per hour, jumped the curb, and crashed into a telephone pole. His Acura sedan was totaled, but he miraculously emerged without any visible signs that he'd been in a wreck. Well, except one. When the driver's side airbag deployed, the Acura logo on it transferred to the palm of Malcolm's hand. He thought it was "kind of a cool tattoo, TBH," and it even stung like fresh ink.

His mother insisted they go to the ED, but Malcolm wasn't bleeding or in any pain. He was also late for tennis practice, so instead, he asked her to drive him to the courts.

"I played the best match of my life. Nothing hurt, and I felt like I was superhuman or something," Malcolm told me, his face lighting up.

I stared at him in amazement. "You went and played tennis right after that?"

He nodded vigorously. "Yeah, and I didn't get tired even though we played for three hours straight. I showed the guys my Acura tattoo, and they were like, 'dude, that's awesome.' I went to dinner, went to bed ... I felt amazing."

When Malcolm woke up the next morning, though, *everything* hurt. His head, his neck, his wrists ... and Malcolm realized that he couldn't remember anything that had happened between the time he crashed into the pole and the time he opened the car door to call his mom. Alarmed, she drove him to our clinic right away for an urgent appointment.

After I examined Malcolm and ordered a head CT, I explained that his post-traumatic amnesia indicated a concussion. I reviewed the importance of rest and close symptom monitoring over the next several weeks, subject to change based on what his CT showed. His mother confirmed that she understood the treatment plan and the "red flags" (confusion, persistent or worsening headache, nausea and vomiting, or decreased coordination) that would necessitate a visit to the ED. I gave Malcolm a letter excusing him from tennis practice and asked what kind of "injection" his chief complaint referred to.

"Oh yeah, can I have an EpiPen for when I go back to tennis practice?" he asked earnestly.

His mother looked at him oddly. "You don't use an EpiPen, Malcolm. You're not allergic to anything."

"I was wondering what happens when you inject yourself with one," he continued.

I, too, was confused by Malcolm's question. I explained that if a person has an anaphylactic reaction to something, like bee stings, the airway muscles swell up and make it hard to breathe. Injecting an EpiPen, so named because it contains epinephrine, relaxes those muscles and keeps the heart pumping fast enough so the person has time to get to the ED for treatment.

Malcolm looked thoughtful. "Okay, cool, because I had this idea. I think the superhuman feeling after the car accident was an adrenaline rush, and I read that adrenaline is the same as epinephrine."

"Yes, that's right," I said slowly.

"So, if I inject myself with an EpiPen, I'll get the superhuman feeling again. Can you prescribe me one? I've seriously never played that well."

A small smile crept across my face. "That's an interesting

thought, but unfortunately, we can only prescribe EpiPens for people with serious allergic reactions. It could save their lives. For you, it would just make your blood pressure and heartbeat go up for a few hours."

"How do you come up with this stuff?" Malcolm's mother cried, rolling her eyes. "I thought the concussion was making you confused and I was gonna have to take you to the ER. Let Emily see her other patients and get on with your bad self."

My teenage patients weren't the only ones with interesting stories behind everyday appointment concerns, of course. There's a joke in family medicine that the real reason a patient comes in isn't revealed until the end of the visit. It's the one that bursts forth when we have one hand on the doorknob and are telling the patient we'll see him or her in six months.

"Hey, Emily, you got any men's vitamins?" a 53-year-old patient named Mr. Fitzgerald asked during one such hand-on-the-doorknob moment. I paused and turned around.

"No, we don't have any vitamin samples since they're available over the counter. Are you worried that some of your levels are low?" Mr. Fitzgerald had come in for seasonal allergies. We hadn't discussed vitamins, but I was happy to.

He laughed nervously. "No, you know ... how should I say it ... not vitamins. Something that would help me perform better for the missus."

"Like Viagra?" I clarified.

"Yeah, yeah!" he responded enthusiastically, looking relieved that he wasn't the one who had to say it out loud.

I bit my lip. "I'm sorry to say we don't have any samples of Viagra, either. It always runs out as soon as it hits the door."

"Well, gimme a call if you get more in," Mr. Fitzgerald replied, jumping to his feet. And with that, he mumbled goodbye and disappeared around the corner quicker than a sample box of Viagra.

CROSSING THE LINE

In some ways, my sworn duties to patients were not unlike marriage vows. I cared for them "for better, for worse, for richer, for poorer, in sickness and in health, until death do us part." I celebrated their joys and personal successes, and comforted them in times of worry, sorrow, or illness. Regardless of whether a month or a year had passed, my reunion with many patients was warm, familiar, open.

One evening, I opened Facebook to see a friend request from a patient, Mr. Murphy. His profile picture showed him with two adorable little boys in T-ball uniforms. They looked like his mini-me's with the same vibrant blue eyes and megawatt smiles, albeit with a few baby teeth missing. Mr. Murphy himself was a super nice guy who never gave me or anyone in the office any trouble. I paused, then decided against clicking on his photo to see the rest of his profile. Instead, I pressed *deny request* and turned to my own newsfeed.

The following morning, I casually brought up the subject to my colleagues while we waited around in the breakroom for our coffee to brew.

"Do y'all ever get friend requests from patients on Facebook?"

Dr. Ackerman, one of the clinic's physicians, nodded. "I ignore the request, and they usually get the message. I find that if I flat out decline it, they act like I personally rejected them and get their feelings hurt."

Kristine, one of the PAs, admitted, "I took my real name off social media so patients can't find me. Even my real friends have a hard time finding me now, but I don't want to deal with all that."

Dr. Ackerman tossed a plastic stirrer in the trash and looked at me grimly. "I don't know why patients think they need to know about what we do in our personal time. I would never want to be friends with my doctor on Facebook."

"Yeah . . ." I said slowly. "I can't tell if this patient doesn't know, doesn't care, or what. He sent me a friend request last night, after I did his prostate exam yesterday."

Kristine's eyes widened, and she almost spit out her coffee. Dr. Ackerman, meanwhile, murmured with mild bemusement, "You must have been very gentle."

"Good god, that is wrong on so many levels," Kristine exclaimed as we watched him walk away. She hesitated before adding, "What did Matthew say?"

I laughed, and the seriousness in the air dissipated. "Oh, you know how he is. He said, 'I hope you said no; otherwise, I'm going to worry that you're starting to like doing prostate exams.' Then we looked at each other and busted out laughing."

The three of us went about our day, and I didn't think anything more of our conversation. Until, that is, Mr. Murphy sent me a second friend request a few days later. Since my *deny* response apparently wasn't a clear enough message, I took Dr. Ackerman's suggestion and ignored it this time. Much to my dismay, Mr. Murphy eagerly asked me at his next appointment whether I had received it, leaving me no choice but to explain why it was inappropriate for me to accept. (I mean, aside from the potential sexual implications since my finger had been in his anus only earlier that week.)

While mutual trust and respect might feel like a friendship, the patient-clinician relationship is a fundamentally unequal one. V. J. Periyakoil, a clinical associate professor of medicine at Stanford, describes it this way: "Being the doctor is all about having control and wielding power, while being a patient is all about loss of control and feeling vulnerable." Clinicians ask personal questions and gain exclusive knowledge of patient views and behaviors, some of which we may disagree with, or which may be illegal. We perform physical exams and procedures that are sensitive, invasive, and even risky. Other kinds of relationships neither expect nor assume this level of trust. Patients must believe, ethically, that we will do no harm, only what is in their best interests, and legally, that we will protect their confidentiality. Despite the privacy policies that social media platforms tout, these forums are not secure modes of communication. While the American Medical Association lays out general recommendations for appropriate social media use, the UK General Medical Council's warning in *Good Medical Practice* is loud and clear: "When communicating privately, including using instant messaging services, you should bear in mind that messages or other communications in private groups may become public." Messages or posts can easily expose PHI, such as a patient's name, age, photos, birthdate, or contact information.

Mr. Murphy appeared skeptical of my explanation. "I doubt you would stop taking good care of me just because you could see my stuff on Facebook."

"It's complicated," I admitted. I told him about a hypothetical case from school, where a patient tells us he usually has just a couple drinks on weekends and that he doesn't do drugs. At some point in the future, we see photos or comments showing him black-out drunk and using cocaine.

"I don't do cocaine. I'm too old for that," Mr. Murphy joked with a grin.

"That's good to hear," I said, laughing. "But can you see how it might put me in a bad spot? Do I make the patient come in and confront him about it? Because now I know he's at high risk of a heart attack or stroke from cocaine, not to mention sudden death because he mixes it with alcohol. I could do nothing, but what if he ODs and dies? I'm going to have to live with the fact that I didn't try to help him."

Mr. Murphy raised his eyebrows and leaned back. "Wow, that got dark fast. I guess you never know what people do in their personal lives," he remarked.

"Exactly. Please don't take it personally that I didn't friend you."

I had another more selfish reason for not wanting patients to friend me. While I would never have to worry about photos of me snorting cocaine or passing out drunk circulating online, Facebook Memories regularly reminded me how much of my personal life I shared with people I barely knew. I was a shining example of someone who put everything on social media, including my wedding photos and other private pictures of my family, my location (*why* had I thought it necessary to check in to every establishment I stepped foot in?), and cryptic, melodramatic Facebook statuses in college that now made me want to hide under a rock. Still, my posts represented the evolution of my life. I had always cared about what other people thought, so I portrayed myself in ways that I believed would interest them. I dwelled on the intentions behind people's words and actions, and I wanted them to care as deeply as I did. Patients were entitled to cast whatever parts of their private lives that they desired into the public eye; surely, I was, too.

Finally, I couldn't help but think about the time I ran into a physician I worked with at the Dallas Pride Parade. I was with my friends, and Dr. Powell was with his partner (now-husband). We enthusiastically greeted each other and had a great time taking in all the festivities. The following day, Dr. Powell sent me a text. He asked me not to tell our colleagues that I had seen him at the parade because they might not find his "lifestyle" acceptable. I promised and kept my word. Based on general office conversations, all our colleagues already knew anyway and, from what I could tell, always treated him with kindness and respect.

I deleted Dr. Powell's text, but the words were seared into my mind. How despicable that he felt he had to hide his identity when he was expected to be unbiased and accepting of all his patients! How pitiful that he had to worry whether his colleagues (and patients, if they knew) would lose respect for or trust in him, even though he was the same excellent, caring, and knowledgeable doctor he'd always been. To a patient, it was just a friend request after a good experience with a clinician. To us, it could mean a ruined reputation, a future lawsuit, a destroyed identity, and the end of a patient-clinician relationship.

Every so often, other patients required reminders about appropriate patient-clinician interactions as well. One Friday afternoon, an urgent appointment appeared at the bottom of my schedule for a 45-year-old woman with vaginal discharge and itching. I glanced at the time displayed in the corner of my computer screen: 4:45 p.m. Of course. Every clinician knows that symptoms that have been going on for a week or more suddenly become urgent at closing time. Vaginal discharge, in particular, seemed to present this way with uncanny frequency.

Ms. Chandler thought she had a yeast infection, and over-the-counter Monistat cream had reduced the itching somewhat but hadn't gotten rid of the discharge. She wasn't sexually active or especially prone to vaginal infections. However, she had recently finished a course of the antibiotic Augmentin for sinusitis. Her nose had finally stopped producing thick, green mucus and congestion, but then things started getting uncomfortable below the belt.

Based on the history she provided, I still suspected a yeast infection, which is a common side effect of antibiotic medications. A nurse chaperoned me as I proceeded with an exam to exclude other diagnoses. Ms. Chandler's legs were up on either side of my head in the dorsal lithotomy position, and I pushed back the skin of her ample thigh with a gloved hand to inspect the vaginal vault.

Suddenly, I heard the unmistakable click of a smartphone camera. I quickly backed my stool away and sat up straight.

"I'm sorry, what are you doing?"

Ms. Chandler didn't so much as look at me or pause as she typed away on her phone.

"My friend texted and asked what I was doing, so I'm going to send her a picture," she replied matter-of-factly.

Before I could say anything, the nurse quickly stepped in and explained that photos of clinic areas were prohibited to ensure patient privacy.

"I'd appreciate it if you deleted that picture," I added, fighting the urge to snatch the phone from Ms. Chandler and do it myself. "It's easy to accidentally expose confidential patient information, and anyway, I'm sure you can understand that I don't want my picture taken in this setting."

"Don't worry," Ms. Chandler responded, finally looking away from her phone and addressing me. "You can't see your face in the picture."

WHAT DO YOU DO FOR WORK?

While I continued to be firm with patients about professional boundaries, I still hadn't mastered the seamless transition from Emily, PA-C, to Emily, regular human being. When I was in PA school, most people I knew couldn't have cared less; we all had our own things going on. Now that I was a practicing PA, they suddenly seemed very interested in what I did for work.

"Hey Emily, can PAs prescribe steroids?" a friend, Jared, yelled over the music at a Halloween party.

"Yeah, I prescribe them here and there when patients have asthma attacks, or for certain kinds of inflammation."

Jared nodded enthusiastically, which made the powder-blue bonnet tied under his chin bob up and down. He was wearing one of those costumes where he was a baby riding around piggyback on an old lady, and his legs were where her legs would be. His outfit came complete with a diaper and a pacifier.

"Niiiice. You think you can prescribe me some?" Jared shouted.

"Why, what's going on?"

"I'm trying to bulk up. I started working with a personal trainer, and I'm already doing protein smoothies and eating six eggs a day. But something like HGH would really help, you know?" Jared attempted to flex his biceps, forgetting that he was wearing an adult baby fat suit.

I laughed, then trailed off when I realized he was totally serious. HGH, or human growth hormone, was what got athletes kicked out of the Olympics and national sports leagues.

"I prescribe steroids like prednisone and dexamethasone, not the illegal kind," I clarified.

Others were equally interested in my potential as a personal pharmacist. At a wedding reception, a woman and I made small talk while we waited in the buffet line. She had gone to high school with the bride and was now working in Dallas as a successful real estate agent. She was super friendly and outgoing, and I liked her right away.

"What do you do for a living?" she asked me.

"I'm a physician assistant. I work in a family practice clinic."

Her eyes grew wide with excitement, as if I had just reported that my occupation was "genie, currently granting wishes."

"What are the chances!" she exclaimed. "I was actually planning to find a doctor soon. My friend gave me two of her Adderall the other day, and it changed my life. I had insane energy and I got *so* much work done. That probably means I have ADD, right, since Adderall worked for me?" She searched my face for signs of confirmation, her shimmery pink eyeshadow glinting in the glow of the buffet table lamps.

"It's possible," I said carefully, "although most people feel more energy when they take Adderall. It's a stimulant, like caffeine, so it speeds things up."

The woman shook her head intently. "Yeah, but it was like day and night for me. Can you write me a prescription? It's *so* crazy that I ran into you here." She executed an impressive over-the-top eyeroll.

I looked down and busied myself with grabbing a dinner plate and utensils from the buffet table. "I can't exactly prescribe anything for you since you're not my patient—"

"I mean, I won't tell if you won't," she returned, raising her eyebrows slyly.

"—but you could always become a new patient at our clinic.

We can test you for ADD and figure out the best treatment for you." I smiled and shrugged apologetically. I probably should have just said no, but I guess I thought I was letting her down gently.

She didn't take the hint. "Can't you just diagnose me here? I don't know why they make this stuff so hard to get. It's not like people are shooting up on Adderall. With all the people who have ADD out there, it should be over the counter by now. Anyway, it was nice meeting you." She flipped her auburn waves over her shoulder and extended her plate toward the waiter serving the Tuscan chicken.

I bit my tongue. If only she knew about the patients I'd seen who had, in fact, injected Adderall. One man came in with his hand so infected and disfigured I thought it was going to have to be amputated. He was sweating bullets, shivering, and screaming like he was possessed while three different nurses attempted IV access for antibiotics. Heroin and Adderall had destroyed most of the man's veins, even the larger ones in his neck and groin. The crazy part? He had never even had a prescription for Adderall; it just happened to be the most recent drug he got his hands on and ignited the infection.

Another patient had created a hole in the septum of her nose, the fleshy piece on the inside, after initially snorting Adderall and then progressing to cocaine. She had come in for a completely unrelated reason (leg pain, maybe?) and I would never have known except that she had a nosebleed in the middle of the appointment. Fifteen minutes and half a box of tissues later, I looked inside her nose with an otoscope and found much more than just an irritated blood vessel. She was how I first learned that Adderall and cocaine were in the same scheduled drug class. Both stimulants could cause sudden death, heart attack, and stroke, and it was easy for people to abuse and become addicted to them. No way was Adderall going to be over the counter in our lifetimes.

With surprise and concern, I realized that, whereas I had once felt useful and flattered that people saw me as a trusted medical source, I was steadily growing weary of fielding every little question that was remotely medical-related. People learned I was a PA and inevitably asked for prescriptions, medical advice, and work excuses when they weren't sick but wanted a day off. The sky was the limit. I didn't hear them immediately asking the guy who worked in IT about the IT issue they were having. Medicine was my passion, but I was more than just my job! After work, I wanted to talk about anything *but* work. Instead, I often felt like a monkey with a prescription pad or like I was on Medical Jeopardy. It didn't seem normal for a PA to feel annoyed or resentful when everyday people asked for help. Was something wrong with me? Had I chosen the wrong career?

THE HAYN BUG

Whenever I shared these fears with my husband, Matthew, he would nobly keep me from completely spiraling away into the clouds of self-doubt.

"You're the most caring and empathetic person I've ever met. That's why you're a good PA," he'd say.

He'd cite my response to the Hayn Bug as proof of my unwavering commitment to those in need. Pronounced "Hane" and short for our last name, Haynie, the Hayn Bug is Matthew's scientific terminology for when he catches a cold. Thankfully, this isn't often, because he pulls out all the stops. Normally strong, energetic, and independent, Matthew behaves like he is on death's doorstep at the first sign of sniffles. He grabs an armful of fuzzy blankets and either wraps himself up like a human burrito or piles them on until every inch of his body is buried under a foot of linen. In a muffled voice, he despondently rasps, "Baby, I don't think I'm gonna make it," and I tenderly hand him medicines to ease his symptoms. At my suggestion, he will take a hot bath, only to send me GIFs of a cartoon character digging his own grave, jumping in, and placing a tombstone on top of the mound of dirt that reads "ME." Then, it's back to bed. He whimpers, "Emily, I think I'm dying," as I stroke his hair and reassure him that he'll recover from this cold. The next day, he accepts my offerings of soups and hot beverages, croaking between sips, "If I die, remember I want a Viking burial . . ."

Despite his Oscar-worthy performance any time the Hayn Bug strikes, Matthew always predictably resists one place with every fiber of his being: the doctor's office.

"You're my doctor," he insists when I recommend making an appointment. "Make me better, Dr. Emily."

One year, after two weeks of this, I gave Matthew an ultimatum: he had to see someone other than "Dr. Emily." I could barely function at work after sleepless nights listening to his coughing and lying next to him while he turned like a rotisserie chicken under the covers. After protesting like I was asking him to make an appointment for a root canal without anesthesia, Matthew finally agreed. A few days later, I sat silently in the exam room while he downplayed his symptoms to his doctor: "Yeah, I've been coughing some."

I wanted to laugh and scream at the same time. *Some?!* He'd been coughing all night, every night, for two straight weeks like he had the plague! He was singlehandedly supporting Halls with his cough drop purchases (I never even knew they made packs of eighty), and his throat and ribs were still sore. We both had bags the size of small countries under our eyes from the lack of sleep.

I made a mental note to take a photo of our bedroom next time as evidence for the doctor. Matthew's nightstand currently looked like a cough drop wrapper graveyard, interrupted only by the occasional Sudafed or Tylenol pill. The trashcan looked like a mad scientist had mixed all kinds of potions and discarded the empty bottles: Chloraseptic throat spray, a greasy jar of Vicks VapoRub, and a container of "sizzurp," an old prescription of Phenergan with codeine that Matthew guzzled like it was the elixir of immortality. I'd have to get footage of when he faded each evening, whispered, "This is the end," and huddled next to me, barely visible under all the blankets.

I could have kissed the doctor who saw Matthew that day and prescribed antibiotics for his bacterial sinusitis. The Hayn Bug had finally been conquered. Well, at least until Hayn Bug 2.0 made an appearance.

BORDERLINE

Ms. Delier, a woman with borderline personality disorder, saw me sporadically. Despite her other chronic conditions of high blood pressure, high cholesterol, and osteoarthritis in both knees, BPD was the only one that cast a shadow over every aspect of her life.

BPD is characterized by "instability of interpersonal relationships, self-image and affects, and marked impulsivity," according to the Diagnostic and Statistical Manual of Mental Disorders (DSM). Ms. Delier had summarized her youth as simply: "my parents just couldn't deal with me." She had run away from home several times, started smoking cigarettes and pot, had her first abortion at age thirteen, and dropped out of school. Her parents had responded to her behavior by kicking her out of the house.

By the time we met in her 30s, Ms. Delier had been fired from numerous jobs for absenteeism or for getting into arguments with coworkers and bosses. She had very few girlfriends and admitted that boyfriends were often physically abusive. She frequently felt empty inside and cut or burned her own skin "to feel something." She'd had at least five more abortions ("I've lost count") and struggled with cigarettes, alcohol, and drugs, prostituting herself for them or stealing whenever she ran out of money. Ms. Delier's interactions with her parents remained unpredictable and chaotic, although still existent.

Sometimes, I wondered if ours was her only stable relationship. I was a reliable, familiar face, someone who continued to listen, even when those outside the walls of the clinic seemed to turn their backs on her. I did not chastise Ms. Delier for noncompliance, despite her undeniably sporadic requests to refill daily prescription medications. I hid my disappointment when she relapsed after one of her many attempts to quit using. People with BPD often have feelings about others that shift quickly; Ms. Delier could idolize me one moment and feel that I betrayed her the next. If I lost her trust, I'd also lose the opportunity to care for her health entirely.

Interacting under the guise of acceptance wasn't easy for me, by any means. I saw quite clearly why Ms. Delier's past psychiatrists and other clinicians had refused to continue care. My patience, too, frayed when I was on the receiving end of the manipulative and oppositional behaviors they described in their notes. Establishing patient rapport sometimes felt impossible. There is no cure for personality disorders, and while Ms. Delier at least appeared to accept her diagnosis, engaging with her BPD was nevertheless trying.

Then, one day, Ms. Delier came to me with a request no patient had ever made before (or since).

"If I tell you something, it stays between you and me, right?" she asked cautiously.

"Yes, everything you tell me is confidential unless you're about to harm yourself or someone else. Then, legally I have to report it," I responded.

"No, I'm not going to hurt anyone." Ms. Delier unzipped her purse and handed me a bottle of Tylenol from it. "You can open it."

I unscrewed the cap and immediately saw pills of all shapes, colors, and sizes. Definitely not Tylenol. I could feel Ms. Delier's slate-gray eyes on me as she waited for my reaction, and with her permission, I emptied the bottle into the palm of my hand. I recognized several Xanax bars, Oxy tablets, and a variety of muscle relaxers. There were also numerous generic, unmarked pills. In the ensuing silence, Ms. Delier admitted she had bought these prescription medicines and illicit drugs from strangers, or pilfered pills from family members. She never sold or gave any away.

I stared at the pills wordlessly, barely registering what she was saying. *What am I supposed to do with these? Why is she showing me her stash? Is she about to pull out an 8-ball of coke next?*

"Do you have other bottles like this at home?" I asked finally, careful to appear curious rather than accusing.

"Just these ones with the meds you give me," Ms. Delier replied, fishing two orange prescription bottles out of her purse. "I don't ever sell or give them away, either," she added. *I'm sure no one's looking for blood pressure or cholesterol pills on the black market,* I wanted to say. Instead, I asked her how many pills she was taking in any given day.

Ms. Delier shook her head. "I don't take them." She paused and corrected herself. "I mean, I did take them, but not for a couple months now. I just keep them on me, and it calms me down just knowing they're there. It's like my mind won't stop otherwise and I have this constant urge to get more…"

She trailed off, clearly conflicted, before speaking again. "I don't take the pills because I'm scared I'll OD one day and die. Can you get rid of them for me?"

I stared at her, stunned. Whatever I thought she was about to say after showing me her stash, it wasn't that.

"Of course I will," I responded as I tried to hide my surprise. Ms. Delier watched as I carefully poured the assortment of pills back into the Tylenol bottle.

"You're not mad?" she asked, looking uncertain.

"I'm relieved, actually. I don't want you to overdose, either, and most people would never be able to do what you just did."

For a time after that appointment, I felt proud. So many clinicians had thrown up their hands in defeat and passed

Ms. Delier and her insufferable borderline off to psychiatry or psychology. But I had persevered in my attempts to be a stable relationship. She trusted me, and that may have saved her life.

And then, suddenly, it hit me. I had somehow made myself the hero, but that was absurd. Ms. Delier had BPD, and there was no cure. I wasn't even trained to provide the first line treatment for it, which was behavioral therapy, so I wasn't meant to fix her problems. I had merely been allowed an occasional glimpse into her private, often painful, world, and happened to bear witness when she made a momentous decision. Throughout all those appointments, I had never considered how distressing BPD was for the patient. I hadn't saved her; *she* had outsmarted her own demons.

A MOTHER'S GRIEF

I was startled when I entered an exam room one morning; I had been taking care of Ms. Ross for years, but I barely recognized her. In place of her normally bright demeanor, tears streamed steadily down her ashen, swollen face. The entire neckline of her shirt was wet, but she did not notice. Alarmed, I handed her a box of tissues and pulled up a chair beside her that was usually reserved for patients' family members.

Trembling, Ms. Ross hoarsely stammered out in barely a whisper that her 16-year-old son, Tyler, had committed suicide.

Her whole body felt like it was in shock. Tyler had never seemed depressed and neither she, her husband, nor their younger son knew he had been struggling. He had not left a suicide note, and there were so many questions she did not have the answers to. Ms. Ross had recently learned information that suggested Tyler's classmates may have bullied him in school and on social media. Just like all the kids his age, Tyler was always on his cell phone. They never saw him do anything more than watch TikTok videos or take a selfie for the Be Real app.

When Ms. Ross and her husband talked to Tyler's teachers and his classmates' parents to find out more about the circumstances surrounding his death, they were shocked and hurt further by the secrecy. The kindest of friends suddenly turned icy and clammed up. Others denied that Tyler had encountered any bullying and insisted he had been well-liked. Tyler did have several close friends that Ms. Ross was aware of, and though they were clearly distraught at his suicide, she sensed that no one was telling her the full story. Her head swirled with all the contradictory and missing information. She wept for her son's hidden pain. She wept for her life without him, the light extinguished from it forever.

Ms. Ross thought her husband seemed to be handling Tyler's death better than she was. Although he talked less at home, he was still able to go to work and take care of things, including their younger son. For her, though, life had stopped the moment she found out Tyler was gone. She had tried to return to work after one week of bereavement leave but could not concentrate on anything, nor sit at her desk for longer than a few minutes without going to the bathroom to cry. Her boss had reduced her hours and allowed her to work in the privacy of her home. He was very supportive; he was the one who had encouraged her to see me.

I referred Ms. Ross for counseling and had frequent follow-ups with her over the next several months. Antidepressant medications helped her sleep but made no difference in the pervasive sadness that weighed her down every moment she was awake. She felt that no one, not even her husband, would ever understand her pain. Anxiety and paranoia about whether kids had bullied Tyler and driven him to suicide plagued her. Ms. Ross could not accept that she would never know what had led him to choose this ending. Things did not have to be this way; Tyler would still be here if only he had asked for help. If only she had been a better, more observant mother. Did she even deserve to still be here when she had failed her child?

Concerned about the survivor's guilt that had emerged in the wake of an unspeakably tragic death, I encouraged Ms. Ross to honor Tyler's memory in meaningful ways—to never let him, or what he meant to the world, disappear. She ultimately decided to participate in the Out of the Darkness Overnight Walk, in which people gather at sunset and walk over sixteen miles until sunrise. Walkers emerge out of the darkness to stand in solidarity, honor those who have died by suicide, and raise money and awareness to prevent future suicides. Ms. Ross also started an organization to prevent bullying on social media, and in recent years, I heard about it on the radio.

Still, nothing would ever bring her son back.

HLF

Ms. Berry, a longtime patient of our clinic, came in one morning for newly diagnosed atrial fibrillation. A cardiologist had confirmed the dangerous arrhythmia with an event monitor, but Ms. Berry was adamantly opposed to treatment. At seventy years old, she took just one prescription medication for high blood pressure and prided herself on her health.

"Ms. Berry, your repeat ECG today still shows AFib," I told her. "I agree with your cardiologist; starting a medication is a good idea."

Ms. Berry frowned as she stared at the squiggly forms on the printed ECG tracing.

"I don't know, Emily. I just don't want to take any medicines if I don't have to. I don't want to become dependent on them."

I smiled politely. This was one of the most common responses I encountered. Patients resist or reject medicines, ironically bargaining instead with those who had made it their life's work to learn this complicated discipline. The "art" of medicine was incorporating both the current evidence and the patient's personal values to plant the seeds of change. Providing facts and information alone, I had learned, did not lead to action.

I shifted in my seat and straightened my posture as I contemplated the path forward.

"Ms. Berry, you always make the final decision," I began.

"You've done so much already to lower your risk of heart attack and stroke by remembering your blood pressure medicine every day, eating well, and being active." Ms. Berry sat up a little straighter herself.

"Thank you," she said, looking pleased.

"But I'm here to make sure we look at the whole picture. These palpitations and dizzy spells are telling you something isn't right. That's why you went to the heart doctor; you were listening to your body. AFib is a new cardiac risk factor for you. It can cause you to have a stroke, and I don't want that for you."

Ms. Berry listened in silence and fidgeted with the thin gold rings on her left hand. The younger me would have immediately gone on and presented my most convincing case for treatment, but I said nothing and let her make the next move.

Finally, Ms. Berry looked up at me. "What are my options?" she asked. I smiled appreciatively and explained that we could do nothing and, because AFib won't go away on its own, accept that she may have a stroke. We could reset her heartbeat with an ablation, but her cardiologist didn't think she was a candidate. Or we could start medication to proactively prevent a stroke.

I paused to let this sink in. "I understand not wanting to take another medicine—it's human nature. I bet the majority of clinicians don't want to start patients on medicines if they don't have to. We constantly weigh the potential benefits against the potential risks."

Ms. Berry rubbed one of her temples wearily.

"Would I have to take the medicine every day?" I nodded.

"One pill a day, just like your blood pressure medicine. Blood thinners can have serious side effects, so we'll need to watch for those. But otherwise, you'll keep on living your life. Take your walks, cook, do your gardening."

Ms. Berry appeared thoughtful and started to ask a question.

Suddenly, there was a wail in the hallway followed by a thud and a sharp knock at the door. I excused myself to crack it open.

"Anna fell," a nurse whispered to me through the gap. I suspected there was more to the story as I opened the door slightly wider and saw Anna, the clinic's insurance specialist, writhing on the carpeted hallway floor.

"I'm so sorry, wait here for me," I apologized to Ms. Berry, who looked terrified.

"Go ahead, I'll be fine. Oh my god," she murmured.

"Get Dr. Mullins," I instructed the nurse as I closed the door behind me and knelt next to Anna. I tapped Anna on the shoulder and called out her name a couple of times like the actors do in CPR training videos. I tried to remain calm as I reminded myself of the ratio of breaths to compressions.

Eerie, rhythmic, unintelligible sounds issued from Anna's throat as her mouth twisted involuntarily. Her hands were balled into fists over her chest, her pupils were unfocused and moved side to side, and her body shook in an uncoordinated fashion. To my relief, she was breathing and had a pulse. There were no signs of injury or bleeding. The nurse returned with a box of the clinic's emergency supplies and looked at me helplessly as I removed various equipment.

"I already called 911. Do we start CPR?" she asked.

"No, she has a pulse and she's breathing. Let's turn her on her side. Did anyone see what happened?"

"She got written up because she was late for the second time this week. She got upset and started yelling, then dropped to the ground and refused to get up." The nurse had a flair for the dramatic, so I wasn't sure how much I could believe her version of the story. She helped me move Anna's legs into a kickstand position, and I did a brief neurological exam and checked her vital signs. Anna's oxygen levels were normal, but her heart rate and breathing were increased. To my relief, EMS and Dr. Mullins—one of the physicians in our clinic—appeared around the corner.

As EMS strapped her to the gurney, Anna stopped making audible sounds and shaking. Her eyes were still open, but she didn't look like she was responding to anything in her environment.

"Glad she's their problem now," Dr. Mullins said as we walked back to our offices. "Looks like a classic case of HLF. We used to see it all the time in the ED."

"HLF?" I repeated. There were so many medical acronyms, and my memory came up with nothing.

"Hysterical Latin Female," Dr. Mullins replied matter-of-factly before hanging up his white coat and leaving for lunch. I stared wordlessly after him, dumbfounded.

A few days later, Anna saw me for a follow-up visit from the ED, and we reviewed her discharge diagnosis together: acute seizure due to alcohol withdrawal. I was beyond surprised. I never saw her drink alcohol, even at staff events and parties. I had never smelled alcohol on her breath and never had a reason to question her work product. I wondered at my own perceptiveness: *what else had I missed?*

After Anna cried in the privacy of the exam room, we discussed her triggers, social situation, and current willingness to quit drinking. I referred her to a psychologist who specialized in substance use disorders and who was comfortable communicating with Spanish-speaking patients. How quickly a clinician's conclusion of "HLF" could have changed Anna's trajectory of care! Anna might not have received lifesaving treatments for her seizures in the ED, or subsequent therapy to help her quit drinking. Seizures are among the most dangerous effects of alcohol withdrawal; in severe cases, they cause permanent brain damage or death. People struggle as it is to overcome alcohol misuse or addiction. A strong, nonjudgmental support team is critical for recovery.

Over the next few weeks, I thought a lot about Anna and HLF. Health inequity already has a tremendous impact on Hispanic/Latinx Americans, who are wildly underinsured compared to White Americans. In 2022, one out of every five to six Hispanic/Latinx people under the age of 65 reported that they had no health insurance coverage at all. Even those with insurance sought care less often because of language barriers, clinic hours that conflicted with their work hours, and lack of transportation and nearby health clinics. And because they thought healthcare professionals would write them off. With clinicians spouting diagnoses like "HLF" as if they were legitimate, it wasn't hard to see why.

A 2019 article in *Physician's Weekly* reported that Hispanic/Latinx patients were 25 percent less likely than White patients to receive medication for acute pain in the ED. Other studies, including one in the *Journal of the American Medical Association (JAMA)* regarding pain treatment for patients with acute traumatic injuries, show similar findings. I wondered if the ED clinicians assumed, like Dr. Mullins had, that Hispanic/Latinx patients were dramatic or that their perceptions of pain were less valid. Racial bias undeniably perpetuates health inequities.

The only "positive" thing Anna's seizure achieved was that Ms. Berry reconsidered treatment for AFib while she sat alone with her thoughts in the exam room. She called her cardiologist from the room and made an appointment for the following week. I provided her with medication samples, which she promised to start the same day, and reviewed the possible side effects. Ms. Berry did not know exactly what had transpired in the hallway, but her initial thought was that someone was dying. She wasn't ready to go that way.

PEDOBUG

Even as I grew into my identity as a PA, my identity as an Asian PA was still a sore point. One patient in particular stoked my initial misgivings and confused thoughts into outright inner turmoil. Thankfully, he represented the extreme: a patient with a persistent and morbid fascination with my ethnicity who was undeterred by both unspoken and explicitly stated rules of professionalism.

Mr. Peterson was a heavy-set white man in his late fifties with a mop of graying brown curls, a bulbous nose, excess skin under his chin, and crumbling, gray fingernails. Without fail, either his chest hair or his gut was visible from his gaping shirt. The first time he met me, he told me he used to live in the Bay Area, "or as I call it, 'Little Asia.'" He was interested in all Asian people but found "Chinese women particularly sensual." That was the day the nickname "The Pedobug" was born. I had never referred to any of my patients with nicknames, but my mind went straight to two things that I found repulsive: pedophiles and bugs.

Larry Peterson
58yo M
Chief complaint: Right foot pain

I groaned after I scanned the schedule on my computer one morning.
"Oh no."

"What is it?" my coworker, Katie, asked.

"The Pedobug is here. He's this older creepy guy who told me he has a fetish for Asians."

She made a face. "Yechh. Good luck, then."

I heaved a sigh of resignation in response, dragged my feet to the exam room door, and knocked.

"Nobody's home," a man's voice called.

I turned the door handle to find the Pedobug laid across the exam table like a Roman stretched across a chaise at Bacchanalia. His Polo shirt was unbuttoned, revealing a shag carpet of curly chest hair and a potbelly. His small, wiry glasses were slightly askew; he had probably flopped down on the table right before I came in, which was unnecessary to begin with since every room had a chair.

"Hi Emily, come on in," the Pedobug said as he made a grand, sweeping gesture with his arm.

"Good to see you, Mr. Peterson. I'm going to need you to sit up first."

"Whatever my Oriental lady desires," he responded, making a big show of doing so and adjusting his shirt so that a little more chest hair peeked out. My stomach churned.

"Just Emily will suffice," I said firmly before referring to the computer screen and changing the subject. "Your right foot has been bothering you lately?"

The Pedobug extended a pudgy, grubby foot toward me in reply, and some flakes of skin fell onto my lap.

"It's my big toe," he said, pointing. "It was fine yesterday and when I woke up, it looked like this."

I glanced down at the swollen, red lump, and eyed his other toes and left foot for comparison. No other redness, swelling, deformity, or signs of trauma.

"Have you ever had gout?" I asked.

He shook his head. "Never."

"And you didn't stub your toe on anything yesterday, or drop something on your foot?"

"No. It was literally normal when I went to bed."

I slipped on a pair of gloves and placed my palm gently beneath the Pedobug's foot to keep it steady as I examined it. I knew clinicians who examined patients' feet with bare hands, but some feet out there were *nasty*. The Pedobug's were no exception. His toenails, though surprisingly clear, looked like talons because they were so long. Curly hairs sprouted from the tops of his toes in random places, like plants searching desperately for sunlight. There was some dark lint between several of his toes—at least, I think it was lint.

"Mr. Peterson, try to move your big toe for me," I instructed. He attempted unsuccessfully; the swelling was too severe. I rested the back of my hand against his toe, which felt like a warm stovetop. An indication of inflammation.

"Don't worry, I can't feel anything," the Pedobug remarked, watching me intently. "I found some old hydros from my back surgery and took them before my appointment." I pressed on the metatarsophalangeal joint at the base of his big toe, and The Pedobug nearly levitated off the table.

"Yiiiikes," he cried out. "Never mind, I felt that!"

"Sorry, Mr. Peterson, I had to check for tenderness. This looks like gout to me."

I explained the treatment plan, including blood tests to check his uric acid level and kidney function; anti-inflammatory medication; and avoidance of triggers like meat, fish, beer, and dehydration.

"Let us know how your toe is in a couple of days," I told him as I handed him his shoes. "The anti-inflammatory should work quickly, and by then we'll have your bloodwork back. I don't expect anything exciting."

"What I wouldn't give to see your feet out of those shoes," the Pedobug replied, staring at my shoes and apparently oblivious to everything I had just said. "I bet you have those dainty little Asian feet."

I stood up immediately and didn't even bother to hide my disgust.

"We're not talking about my feet," I said sternly. "Give us a call in a couple of days and let us know if you're better." *You perv.*

Katie swiveled around in her chair when I returned to our office.

"So? How did it go?" she inquired.

I snorted. "Well, the appointment ended with him saying I had dainty little Asian feet and with me feeling like I was on OnlyFans. So, I'd say, 10 out of 10," I replied sarcastically. I sat back down at my desk and tried to reset my focus before my next patient. The Pedobug's Asian fascination was an extra distraction I didn't need in a job that constantly required my energy, attention, and clinical judgment. It had gotten harder to remain calm and professional over progressive visits, and I had let him ruffle my feathers today.

I saw The Pedobug for several more years. I continued to deflect his references to my "honey skin tone" or "almond-shaped eyes." One day, I was surprised to see that he was on a physician's schedule instead of mine. *He's finally gotten the message that I'm not tolerating his BS and weird Asian fetish,* I thought with satisfaction. The real reason, I found out, was that The Pedobug turned sixty-five and transitioned to Medicare for his health insurance. PAs were not contracted with Medicare at our clinic. I never thought I would say this, but *thank you, Medicare!*

IT'S BEEN A LONG DAY, TO SAY THE LEAST

I remember how I once crouched behind a check-out desk after an angry patient threatened to "get my gun out of my truck and shoot this place up." To this day, I still don't know the circumstances that prompted his statement, only the terror he incited. After the man slammed the door on his way out, someone had locked it and called the police. Blissfully ignorant, I had accompanied a patient to check-out when an unexpected scuffle of activity greeted us in the lobby. People were running in every direction, and the patient and I followed the receptionist's frantic instructions and obediently lowered ourselves to the ground behind the desk, huddling next to strangers. As the patient texted someone from her cell phone, I remembered that my phone was locked in my desk drawer. I usually didn't keep it on me because I didn't want it to ring or buzz during appointments. My heart pounded while I tried to soothe my patient and to not think about what was going to happen to us.

A tense ten minutes followed. Someone said he did not believe the patient and that he was just trying to scare us. Someone else asked if the glass door and windows that made up the entire front wall of the clinic were bulletproof. A few staff members debated exiting through the back doors to where their cars were parked, with each of us loading as many patients into our vehicles as could fit. This idea was quickly extinguished; the manager had locked all external and internal clinic doors to reduce access to potential victims.

As the minutes went by and nothing happened, people relaxed slightly, and someone even joked that the man must have forgotten where he had parked. The police arrived and played the clinic's security camera footage: the man had gotten in his truck and driven away, and they had reason to believe he was not coming back. An officer would remain nearby to patrol in case the situation changed.

After further discussion, the manager unlocked the front door and told us to go back to work and to reassure the patients. Forget about that nervous, sick feeling I had in my stomach five minutes ago when I thought this might be how I spent my last moment on earth, hiding behind a desk and unable to even text my family that I loved them. Patients were waiting and there was work to do.

TWO HONEY BUNS OR TWO ALMONDS?

I had been pleasantly on schedule the day Ms. Toth came to see me for a weight loss follow-up. The EMR showed that she had checked in early; as it approached ten minutes past her scheduled appointment time, however, she was still not in an exam room. I made my way toward the medical assistants' workstation to verify that they hadn't overlooked her in the waiting area.

As I rounded the corner, I saw what the holdup was. The medical assistants asked all patients to please take off their shoes before stepping on the scale to measure their weight. Ms. Toth was evidently in the process of removing everything else as well. Off came her sweater, belt, purse, and bracelets. She carefully deposited these items in a steadily growing pile before turning at last to face her dreaded foe. Oh, wait. She had forgotten to take off her earrings. Okay, now she was ready.

I had been watching Ms. Toth as if in a trance, and finally turned away to walk back to my office just as I heard her cry out: "What?!"

Ms. Toth wasn't the first patient to engage in such a psychological struggle when approaching the scale, which was, for us healthcare professionals, simply a tool to screen for obesity (and a most primitive one at that). Many patients displayed grim determination, muttering to the scale or shedding belongings in attempts to change a fixed result.

When our appointment started, 21-year-old Ms. Toth sat, dejected, with her back against the wall and her eyes on the ceiling. Her copper-brown hair had partially escaped her ponytail holder, and her belongings were strewn across the exam room counter between jars of tongue depressors and cotton-tipped applicators. She didn't look at me as I sat down and silently reviewed her vitals in the chart: one pound less than last month's reading in our clinic.

"Ms. Toth, tell me what's on your mind," I coaxed.

"One fucking pound," she responded, bitterly emphasizing each word. When she finally met my eyes, she looked like she was about to cry. I reassured her that this was perfectly normal. Weight loss was a slow, gradual process that required difficult changes over the long term. That was why she and I would be meeting often in the first several months until she found a routine that worked for her. We had discussed several potential eating plans at her initial consultation: Weight Watchers, paleo, Atkins... Which one had she decided to go with?

"I've been gluten-free for a whole month! Not even one cheat day!" Ms. Toth lamented.

"Have you ever been diagnosed with Celiac disease?" I asked. This wasn't listed in her past medical history, but I gave her the benefit of the doubt. Records were often incomplete or not up to date.

"No."

"Did you stop eating gluten because it was giving you stomach problems?"

"No," Ms. Toth snapped. "My friend and me just wanted to be healthier, so we both started a gluten-free diet."

"Okay, I think I know what we can do," I said as I contemplated the right words. It was an easy mistake, really. Ms. Toth had interpreted *diet* the way the general public did (a way to lose weight), rather than by its medical meaning (what a person normally eats and drinks on a daily basis). Gluten is the main ingredient in wheat. It is only a problem for people with Celiac disease, a serious autoimmune condition: when they eat gluten, it damages their small intestine and increases the risk of cancer and heart disease. Eating foods without gluten—a gluten-free diet—is therefore the medical treatment for Celiac disease. Since Ms. Toth did not have Celiac disease or gluten intolerance, avoiding wheat would make no difference. She would not become healthier, and she would continue to be disappointed if her goal was weight loss.

As understanding crept over Ms. Toth's face, she seemed relieved that the one-pound weight loss did not reflect personal failure.

"I'm glad I found that out now and not a few months from now," she said earnestly. "I would be so mad I'd probably stop trying." She could handle paleo, she said, and she left the appointment sounding hopeful again.

A colleague of mine had once described this disconnect between patients' general knowledge and their understanding of health concepts by saying that "literacy is not health literacy." Like most of my patients, Ms. Toth had completed some form of education. She was literate, intelligent, and interested in her health. Patient education was still necessary, however, because medicine was a specialized subject matter. The near-daily conversations I partook in about obesity and weight loss couldn't be more different from the simulated appointment scenarios my classmates and I had diligently practiced on one another in PA school. Unlike my patients, my classmates all had normal BMIs, specialized knowledge about obesity, and above-average interest in health behaviors. It was impossible to follow the simple directive our professors had distilled weight loss down to: if patients have obesity or obesity-related health conditions, counsel them on diet and exercise. The clinicians I worked with also had widely disparate approaches, which made me wonder if maybe we were all just winging it and relying on our own intuition. I started my own mental list of dos and don'ts beginning with what Ms. Toth had taught me:

DO
Ask patients what diets they have tried in the past and personalize weight loss plans.

DON'T
Assume patients understand everything.

Another one of my patients, Ms. Robinson, threw a little twist into our weight loss conversation. She had lost over 100 pounds in the six months following a lap band surgery, and then dropped an additional thirty pounds by one year. When her high blood pressure, acid reflux, and sleep apnea all improved tremendously as a result, I was able to reduce the doses of her prescriptions and even eliminate some of them. Ms. Robinson was overjoyed about all the things she could now do on her own. She played with her grandkids, cleared out space at home for an artist's studio where she could paint and sculpt, shopped, vacationed with her husband—everything that she desired for a full life. At forty-five years old, she was excited about her future for the first time in many years.

I skimmed Ms. Robinson's log of weekly weigh-ins, which her bariatric surgeon had recommended to help her maintain weight loss. Around fourteen months, Ms. Robinson's numbers had started trending down more slowly. This was not uncommon; people usually lose the most weight in the first one to two years after bariatric surgery. However, the upslope in recent weeks caught my attention because some patients also regain about a third of the lost weight by ten years post-surgery.

"I'm so mad at myself," Ms. Robinson groaned, dismayed. "I can't go back to where I was."

I set the log aside. "You've gone up less than ten pounds, so don't panic. Let's talk about what changed this month."

Ms. Robinson looked down and studied her lap silently before speaking again.

"So, you know how I've just been eating, like, six bites for lunch and dinner? I was doing everything they told me to do: cutting all my food into tiny pieces and chewing slowly so that I won't just be sitting there, staring at my empty plate while everyone else eats. It's just . . . not the same as eating a real meal." She frowned.

"Learning new ways to eat takes a lot of work," I acknowledged, sensing her frustration. "Do you think it would help if you got everyone else at home on board? That way you're not the only one watching how much you eat."

Ms. Robinson squirmed. "Well . . . I kind of figured out a solution. If I jump around after a few bites, I can move the food past the lap band without throwing up. That's why I gained weight—I'm eating more." She shrank back as she said this, like a child afraid that I was going to strike her. Indeed, it was important for Ms. Robinson's improving health and activity status to discourage the behavior and suggest different ones as she navigated a complicated relationship with food and eating. But I couldn't help thinking, perhaps I should give her credit for being honest with me . . . or at least for her creativity.

DON'T
Assume patients I understand everything.

In his mid-fifties with slightly graying hair, Mr. Ramsey was reading a magazine on monster trucks when I walked in. He was a hefty man and an impressive gut hung over the waist of his jeans. He eyed me suspiciously over his reading glasses, and when he did so, the ample skin of his neck pooched under his chin, resembling a rabbit's dewlap.

"So you're the famous Emily, huh," he grunted. "My wife said I had to come see you for weight loss since you've helped her lose fifty pounds. Danielle Ramsey."

I smiled warmly. "Yes, I know Ms. Ramsey! It's wonderful to meet you, too."

Mr. Ramsey didn't return my smile. Crossing his arms, he responded, "Don't get too excited. I don't trust doctors. I just promised her I'd come"—he stretched his arms wide dramatically—"so here I am."

"Fair enough," I said, bringing my energy down a notch so as not to appear too enthusiastic. I started with a few of the more innocuous questions, like when was the last time he saw a doctor ("The only doctor I like is Dr. Pepper.") and what did he like to do for fun ("Fishing, hunting, and anything else where I can get some peace and quiet.") I was surprised by how different Mr. Ramsey's personality was from his wife's. She was bubbly, outgoing, and lighthearted. He had a face of stone in which the frown lines of his mouth seemed permanently etched.

When I told Mr. Ramsey that there was no need to rush anything and that we didn't have to talk about weight loss in our first conversation together, he looked surprised. Apparently, past encounters with healthcare practitioners had inevitably devolved into lectures and critiques about his weight.

"They'd try to put the fear of God in me, like I was going to die the next day if I didn't lose weight," he recalled glumly, taking off his glasses and rubbing his eyes. "I'd come in for something totally unrelated, like an eye infection, and they'd somehow find a way to work it in. It made me want to eat more just to piss them off." A muscle in his jaw tightened involuntarily.

"I'm sorry that happened to you," I said quietly after a moment.

Mr. Ramsey snorted. "They asked me if I'd ever tried to lose weight. Of course I had! You think I wanted to be three hundred pounds? I did Weight Watchers with my wife for a long time, but it got hard because a lot of places don't put points on the menu."

"I know, and it would help a lot of people if they did," I agreed. I usually asked patients about past diets they had tried during the initial consultation, and Mr. Ramsey had inadvertently provided me with some information. I went with it.

"What other things did you try?" I asked casually. Mr. Ramsey furrowed his brow and thought for a moment, although he didn't seem annoyed by the question.

"I did the Subway diet . . . I got sick of those sandwiches, though." He snorted again. "And even sicker when that stuff about Jared came out. I did keto once upon a time, which was great, but my kidney doctor said to stop."

I nodded as I typed this into Mr. Ramsey's chart. Like many patients with hypertension and diabetes, he had chronic kidney disease. The amount of protein in the keto diet might be too hard on his kidneys, which were already damaged, and could cause new problems like gout, kidney stones, and kidney failure.

"And now I'm on the seafood diet," Mr. Ramsey continued.

I tilted my head curiously. "Seafood diet? I haven't heard of that one, but it sounds like something I could get on board with. Can you tell me more about it and what you eat in a typical day?"

For the first time during our appointment, Mr. Ramsey granted me a sly smile.

"Oh, it's simple. When I *see food*, I eat it."

In spite of myself, I laughed. I turned back to the computer and added *seafood diet* to Mr. Ramsey's note, making sure to include quotation marks.

DO
Be thoughtful and sensitive in conversations with patients about weight loss.

DON'T
Take myself too seriously.

One specialist I'd run into occasionally at continuing education lectures described herself as "very blunt" when she counseled patients on weight loss. Dr. Mandell was an endocrinologist who specialized in thyroid and parathyroid disease, and her clinical practice now focused primarily on obesity and weight management. As she put it, "anyone can treat hypothyroidism and hyperthyroidism, and those patients do fine and have a normal life expectancy. People with obesity are the ones who need help so that they don't meet an early death." (Did I say she was very blunt?) Dr. Mandell's counseling methods could purportedly inspire a change of heart in patients who only ate fast food and hadn't exercised since their third-grade PE class.

In a presentation she gave to a group of PCPs, Dr. Mandell explained that extra body fat isn't just about appearance. The American Medical Association designated obesity as a medical disease in 2013 because it increases a person's risk for heart attack, stroke, and type 2 diabetes. The National Cancer Institute also recognizes multiple cancers associated with overweight and obesity, including breast, endometrial, ovarian, kidney, colon, and thyroid cancer. A poster in Dr. Mandell's waiting room boldly announced this fact: "Obesity Begets Cancer."

"As you might imagine, it gets patients' attention," Dr. Mandell said. "They sit in the waiting room wondering about it, and then they ask me during their consultation. People are okay with being obese, but they really don't want to get cancer. It's the perfect way to open the door to that conversation."

Dr. Mandell advised us to be direct with patients about the

importance of treating obesity. We had so little face time with them as it was, and obesity-related diseases waited for no one.

"I don't beat around the bush. I tell patients, 'It's either lose weight or have a heart attack; this is serious.'"

Whew, that's intense, I thought. That would certainly jolt me into action. I'd at least lose some sleep over it. I wondered how her patients reacted.

"This isn't the time to worry about feelings," Dr. Mandell continued sternly. "It's the time to worry about whether they're going to live to see their kids and grandkids grow up. Whether they're going to be able to walk this time next year, or if half their body is going to be paralyzed from a stroke."

A few people in the audience nodded in agreement, and I thought of the youngest patient I'd ever seen who'd had a heart attack. He was eighteen years old and had missed his high school graduation because of it. He had obesity and high blood pressure and had stopped taking his medicine for the latter because he "felt fine" and got tired of taking medicine every day. After the heart attack, he had to take a whole lot more than just one medication. I thought of the young woman I'd seen who'd had a heart attack at age thirty-two. She was overweight, smoked, and rarely exercised. Now, she was also severely depressed after quitting her job, moving back in with her parents, and living in fear of having another attack. Heart attacks are not one and done. Within a year, half of all survivors are hospitalized again with another, and as many as 1 in 10 people die.

Although their lives had changed irreversibly, these two patients were the lucky ones. Many others did not make it out alive. They never had the chance to try different medicines or do cardiac rehab. They didn't have one more appointment where a Dr. Mandell counseled them on weight loss. All that remained of them were grieving loved ones: fatherless and motherless children, childless parents, widowed spouses, and friends left behind.

Many of my patients successfully lost weight after they worked with Dr. Mandell, and her impressive waiting list for new patient appointments proved she was highly sought after. Her style was not for everyone, however. One day, I came across Dr. Mandell's name on a list of recent clinic visits in a patient's chart.

Abcde Powers
30yo F
Chief Complaint: Weight loss

"How did your appointment go with Dr. Mandell?" I asked Ms. Powers. (Her first name, by the way, is pronounced "ab-sid-ee." To my surprise, there were a number of Abcdes in the practice.)

"That's the last time I'll be going to her," Ms. Powers replied sourly. "Her bedside manner is horrible."

I turned away from the computer. "I'm sorry you didn't have a good experience. She can be very blunt; she even says so herself."

Ms. Powers gave me a sarcastic smile. "No, Emily, 'blunt' doesn't cut it. I thought she was going to be happy that I'd lost five pounds since our first appointment. But she just says, 'Only five pounds? You need to be losing five pounds a month.'"

"Don't get discouraged," I implored her. "You're moving in the right direction, and she's going to keep pushing you. That's her brand of tough love."

Ms. Powers squared her jaw. "I told her I was having a hard time losing more, and that I think it's because of my thyroid. She says, 'Because of your thyroid or your mouth?'"

Ouch. I knew that one of Dr. Mandell's favorite mantras was "don't blame your thyroid." Hypothyroidism, or an underactive thyroid gland, is common, and because symptoms may include weight gain, patients frequently point to it as a scapegoat, even when their hypothyroidism is properly treated and hormone levels are normal. But hypothyroidism is hardly the only culprit for weight gain: there's calorie intake, inactivity, stress, poor sleep, genetics, swelling, and medications, among other things. Dr. Mandell thus adamantly discouraged patients from pinning it on existing thyroid disease. Thyroid problems were a convenient and simplistic answer; the biological processes involved in putting on the pounds were far more complex.

When I realized I wasn't going to change Ms. Powers' mind about Dr. Mandell's advice, I moved on to her other concerns. Personally, I still had a lot of respect for Dr. Mandell, who worked tirelessly to involve patients in their own health and instructed them on effective ways to reduce the damaging impacts of obesity. I, too, wanted to be more direct with patients, equipping them with accurate information and a desire to change. But seeing reactions like Ms. Powers', I thought that there had to be a middle ground.

DO
Discuss with patients how common overweight and obesity are, and why it matters just as much as mental, physical, and sexual health.

DON'T
Neglect their emotions.

Since becoming a PA, I'd overheard catchy phrases in public like "she ain't a lady unless she's 280," "I like her thicker than a Snickers," and "your woman can look like a snack, but I want mine to look like Thanksgiving dinner." I wholeheartedly supported vocal appreciation for natural bodies. I didn't want any woman (or man, but go along with the saying) who weighed 280 pounds to feel unhappy with or ashamed of her body.

It was when extra body fat put stress on the woman's frame and she came to me for hip pain that her weight became my concern. When excess weight increased the strain on her heart and lungs, I was responsible for helping her understand the gravity of the situation. When she had prediabetes and obesity, I found it unconscionable not to encourage her to lose weight to prevent full-on diabetes. Obesity-related diseases didn't happen overnight, so I had to look beyond current health status and test results to see the bigger picture. To say it was challenging to navigate the tightrope between encouraging body positivity and effectively communicating the health risks associated with obesity is an understatement.

Acknowledging my own implicit bias was also uncomfortable. Like many people, I incorrectly believed that thin meant healthy. This stemmed from messages and reinforcement over many years by popular culture, family, and finally, PA training. Every magazine and CD album cover I admired as a teenager portrayed a photoshopped celebrity with legs for miles, perfectly airbrushed makeup, and curves in only a couple of places. My parents, who have viewed nutrition, exercise, and weight as a reflection of health for as long as I can remember, grew up in China during the Cultural Revolution. Although they rarely speak of those years because they were fraught with confusion and worry, they recall how all food was rationed, nutritious options were not always available, and snacks like peanuts and sunflower seeds were only sold on special occasions like Chinese New Year. Typical meals included rice or sweet potato. Red meat and fish were available once or twice a month, chicken once or twice a year. Most people were too poor to afford food, and everyone was in the same situation except government officials. In photos, Mom and Dad were always thin because they were hungry. Access to food improved by the time they went to college, but most of their growth was over by then, too.

Mom and Dad took great care to provide my brother and me with filling meals complete with all the recommended food groups. My PA education echoed my parents' convictions: obesity was an epidemic that must be stopped, and losing weight allegedly fell under the same category of "lifestyle changes" as quitting smoking and drinking less alcohol. The messages never wavered or contradicted each other.

One day at lunch, I scrolled through my Facebook news-feed on my phone and paused on a post: "Not one person on *My 600-Lb. Life* was single. Get you that extra honey bun, girl, and gimme two." I'd first come across the reality TV show on TLC at 1:00 a.m. in a hotel room when there was nothing interesting on. Twenty minutes later, I was hooked, and I have to give credit to *My 600-Lb. Life* as an unlikely source of perspective and growth. People allowed camera crews into their homes to document the isolating and disabling effects that severe obesity had on their bodies, daily activities, relationships, and outlooks on life. Despite the show's title, there was no upper limit; some people were 700 or 800 pounds, or as much as 919 pounds. Sometimes, they shopped for and prepared their own meals, suffering cruel stares or comments from strangers at the store. Other times, significant others or family members assisted them.

In one episode, a woman's boyfriend mixes her favorite foods (pizza, ice cream, hot dogs, tacos, etc.) in a blender and pours it through a funnel into her mouth several times a day. For me, eating is one of life's greatest pleasures, and consuming it in liquid form every day would be my worst nightmare. *Why would she choose to live like that?* It turns out the woman had always wanted to be a plus-sized model. More specifically, she wanted to weigh 1,000 pounds. She filmed herself eating on camera, and once the money started coming in from strangers, her boyfriend conceived the idea of funnel-feeding to help her reach her goal weight. The woman relished his attentiveness, and he was more than happy to do it because she was realizing her dream. Her family, although concerned about the effects of severe obesity on her health, nevertheless supported her endeavors because they, too, wanted to see her happy.

In other *My 600-Lb. Life* episodes, people seek help from a bariatric surgeon, and fear of dying due to their weight is a common theme. This was eye-opening for me. Patients I'd seen with severe obesity had never intimated this particular fear, and I thought about how it would feel to hear a clinician say that they needed to eat better and exercise when something far greater weighed on them. I realized that although I wasn't 600 pounds, I shared the basic human desires and some of the psychological struggles of people on the show. My favorite foods were bad for my high cholesterol and encouraged plaque in my blood vessels and a higher risk of heart disease. Yet cravings and emotions regularly defied logic and knowledge, resulting in an internal tug-of-war. Sometimes, I felt guilty because I yearned to be healthy and a role model for my patients, not a hypocrite for counseling them to *do as I say, not as I do*. Any clinician who talks to patients about weight, I think, would benefit and gain new insights from watching *My 600-Lb. Life*.

By no means am I advocating for self-love over health in the context of weighing 600 pounds or more. There is a ceiling, a threshold above which obesity begets cancer and precludes a full life. The more excess weight, the greater the risk of illness, disability, and early death. But we are inadequate as clinicians if we close our minds off to what drives a disease that afflicts so many. It is like giving up on finding a cure for a certain type of cancer because one doesn't exist yet. Just like every other medical condition we treat patients for, a subpar or inaccurate understanding of the causes impedes effective management. Ignoring our implicit biases—or worse, pretending like we don't have any—stunts our capacity for growth and compassion.

What TLC should air alongside *My 600-Lb. Life* is a show on almond moms. Don't know what an almond mom is? Neither did I. Rebecca Walker first used the term positively to connote a woman who was devoted to both her career and her family in her book *To Be Real: Telling the Truth and Changing the Face of Feminism*. In recent years, however, "almond moms" signified something more ominous: mothers with a deep-rooted belief that being thin is an ideal to be pursued at all costs. Not only do they ruminate on their own body image, popular diets, and interpretations of "healthy" eating, but they often impose those same beliefs and behaviors on their children. Rather than promoting self-love and self-worth, they can set their offspring up for lifelong unhealthy relationships with eating. This more negative connotation of "almond mom" arose after an old clip from *The Real Housewives of Beverly Hills* showed former model Yolanda Hadid talking over the phone to her daughter, Gigi Hadid, who was around eighteen years old at the time and also a model.

Yolanda's then-husband, David Foster, tells Yolanda that Gigi is "feeling a little dizzy because she's on that fast" and hands Yolanda the phone.

"I'm feeling really weak. I had, like, half an almond," Gigi says.

Her mother's response? "Have a couple of almonds and chew them really well." Yolanda later defends her words as post-anesthesia gibberish since she had just awakened from a surgery, but plenty of other footage shows that this was not her first time explicitly commenting on Gigi's weight or eating habits.

"Gigi's in charge of her own diet, but to be on your best weight, you gotta make the right choices," she says in one clip. "You can have one night of being bad and then you gotta get back on your diet," she says to Gigi in another. These conversations were as equally painful to watch as the family interactions featured in *My 600-Lb. Life*. Almond moms so idolize a slender frame that they inflict their distorted and unhealthy perspectives on their children, and especially their daughters, in a myriad of ways. They may admonish them when they see them eating, take away their plates before they are full, lock the refrigerator or pantry, force them to do "weigh-ins" at home, and make disparaging comments about their bodies on a regular basis.

Many moms believe they are doing their children a favor because they will not be as loved, successful, or happy if they aren't a size zero. What comes of these messages and behaviors? One in eleven people in the United States has an eating disorder in their lifetime, and over 10,000 people die each year as a direct result, according to the National Association of Anorexia Nervosa and Associated Disorders. It is a sad and unacceptable situation. Parents are usually the adults who are around their children the most during very impressionable years, and whether they want to be or not, they are their role models. It is hard to undo the damage from criticizing a child's weight and appearance, even with time, therapy, and support.

Ultimately, it took years of clinical practice and patient conversations for me to finally grasp that thinness did not equal healthy. Thin people also had type 2 diabetes, osteoarthritis, and cancer. Thin people sometimes had normal bloodwork just weeks before they had a heart attack. A patient might be skinny not because she had self-control and discipline when it came to eating, but because she was exercising constantly and taking laxatives after every meal. My job was to support patients' health, and if they sacrificed it to be thin, then I wasn't doing it successfully.

DO
Find out what my own biases and beliefs are about body weight.

DON'T
Think I ever understand someone else's experience.

A FATHER'S MISFORTUNE

While at Sinclair Family Practice, I came to know a beautiful family. A mother brought her two teenage boys to see me every year for their school physicals, and I celebrated with them when they graduated from high school and went to college. Their stepfather sometimes accompanied them. The boys had been very young when their mother remarried, so now he was simply Dad. He loved the boys fiercely, as if they were his own flesh and blood. He worked hard to provide for them and always supported their dreams. And he was a doting husband who made his wife so, so happy.

One afternoon, the mother came in with both sons. Even as I thought, *What a treat! Both boys are home from college,* the room somehow seemed uncharacteristically devoid of joy and laughter. Seconds later, they revealed the heartbreaking reason for their visit: Dad had been killed in a gruesome accident. When he pulled up to the office parking lot that day, just like he did every day, the automatic gate wouldn't open. He got out of the car to manually lift the gate arm but it still wouldn't budge, so he pressed the button to call security. A line of cars formed behind his as he spoke to someone on the other end.

Suddenly, Dad's car started rolling forward. Employees jumped out from their own cars to help, but it was too late: Dad's car had pinned him against the gate, and he died on impact. The officers and mechanics who arrived suspected that Dad had pressed "brake hold" instead of moving the gear shift to "park." After a certain amount of time, if the brake hold is still on, the driver must press the brake again or brake hold releases. Dad had been outside of the car for a while since he had to call security, and the car had automatically shifted back into "drive."

The sons had been in class when they learned the news, and they couldn't make sense of what had happened. They kept expecting Dad to walk through the door and say that he had missed them since they had last seen one another a month ago. Overcome with disbelief and sorrow, each son gripped one of Mom's hands tightly as sobs racked her body. This was the first time she had left the house since the accident, they told me, and only because they carried her off the living room couch and forced her into the car. I sat with the three of them for some time, listening to the sons' sweet memories of Dad between their tears.

About a year later, the mother informed me that she had been diagnosed with colon cancer. A neurologist had started a workup after an initially innocuous finding of anemia on routine bloodwork, and now the mother was preparing for surgery. She was in her mid-50s, and her colonoscopy had been normal just a few years ago. I remembered how some studies showed that extreme psychological stress, such as the loss of a spouse or a child, increased the incidence of certain cancers. The overall evidence is conflicting, and even the studies that found an association showed only minimal increases, but scientists do know that chronic stress can worsen other health conditions. The theory is that it increases inflammation in the body and weakens the immune system. When people experience profound grief, their habits—like eating, exercising, sleeping, and increased smoking or alcohol use—often change as well. Perhaps this made them more vulnerable to cancer.

As I sat across from the family with its noticeably missing member, I felt a deep ache. Their grief was as fresh as it was a year ago; "time doesn't make it hurt less," they told me. The sons had grown up much sooner than they had needed to when Dad had died. They were forced to once more as they supported Mom through colon cancer. I found myself saying that, although life causes a lot of pain, good things would still happen, too. I wasn't entirely sure I believed this. I couldn't bring Dad back and couldn't take away Mom's potentially fatal illness. But I was desperate to encourage even the smallest sliver of hope. It wasn't blind faith or outright optimism; hope was a life raft. Everyone needs it at some junction, and sometimes it is the only thing that allows us to keep going.

One evening, my cell phone rang while I was on a date with Matthew. I glanced at the screen: Mom. *I'll call her back after we finish dinner*, I thought. After she called two more times and left a voicemail in quick succession, however, I knew something was wrong and called back. She picked up immediately, and I heard sobbing and unintelligible blubbering on the other end.

Alarmed, I said, "Mom, please stop crying. I can't understand anything you're saying."

Between wails, she choked out, "Emily, your dad . . . in the hospital . . . call Eric."

"What! What happened?" My heart leapt into my throat and my stomach turned. My dad and my 13-year-old brother, Eric, had been skiing in Park City, Utah, for spring break. Mom wasn't with them because she had stayed home in Missouri, and I now lived in Texas.

Mom couldn't string two words together to tell me what had happened, so I hurriedly interrupted, "Okay, I'm gonna call Eric now, but I need you to calm down, okay?" I may as well have been speaking another language; she was utterly inconsolable. I promised to call her back, hung up on her sobs, and mouthed 'sorry' to Matthew as I walked out of the restaurant. I called Eric on speed dial.

"Sup," he answered on the second ring.

"Mom said Dad's in the hospital. What happened?"

"Yeah, he broke his leg. At least it's the left one so he can still drive."

I was stunned as to why my brother sounded bored out of his mind while our mother was beside herself. She had made it seem like Dad had died.

"Can he walk?" I asked Eric breathlessly.

"No, he's going to have surgery."

Turns out, while my brother was rippin' and roarin' down a Black Diamond, my 60-year-old dad skied separately down a Blue. While passing over a deceptively small hill, his skis made contact with ice. He leaned a little too hard to keep his balance and went spinning off the path, eventually crashing into a tree and breaking his leg. Unable to stand, Dad radioed for help. After the ski medic located him and an ambulance took him to Park City Hospital, which was a mere ten minutes away, the triage team there recommended transporting Dad to the University of Utah because they were better equipped to handle his complex injury. A second ambulance thus drove him fifty minutes to the latter, with Eric in the passenger seat.

Eric told me the harrowing story as if commenting on the weather. He was mostly bummed that it was only the second day of spring break. He still had a lot more skiing he wanted to do.

"Our rental car's still at the lodge. I don't even know how we're going to get back," he said in a disappointed voice.

"We'll figure that out, Eric," I responded impatiently. "Can I talk to Dad?"

"Nah, I'm in the chapel downstairs. I needed some peace and quiet."

I felt my blood pressure shoot up. "You left Dad by himself

with a broken leg? What is wrong with you! Go back to Dad's room right now so I can talk to him."

Eric groaned. "Ughh, fine. It just got too loud. A ton of doctors kept coming in the room and asking me questions."

Begrudgingly, Eric dragged his feet out of the hospital chapel's serenity and back to the hospital room. Dad's voice sounded small and far away as he recalled the unexpected bump he hit on the slope, the moment of impact, and the blinding pain that followed. He had lain helplessly in the snow for what seemed like an eternity before the ski medic came. He was disoriented because the surrounding grove of trees looked the same in every direction, and he couldn't see or hear any other skiers. He had barely been able to push himself into a sitting position; the snow was deep, and his leg was fractured in two places. My normally strong, stoic father was almost in tears as he described how he did not have any medicine for pain during the bumpy snowmobile ride down the mountain, the fifty-minute ambulance ride, or the leg x-rays in the ED. Thankfully, he had some morphine in him now, so the pain was bearable.

"Let me have you talk to the doctor. I'm starting to feel a little drowsy from the medicine," Dad said to me.

A man's voice came on the other end, quiet but authoritative. "This is Dr. Forshaw."

"Hi Dr. Forshaw, I'm Emily, Andy's daughter. He's getting surgery soon?" The words all ran together and poured out of my mouth like I couldn't stop them.

"Hi, Emily, yes. I'm one of the orthopedic surgeons on Andy's team, and we're about to take him down to the OR now. Surgery should start in about thirty minutes. Andy told me you're a PA?"

"Yes," I answered, pacing.

"That's great. We're going to do an open reduction and internal fixation and put two titanium rods in. Should take about two hours, and then we'll monitor him in recovery."

"Will he be able to walk after surgery?" I asked anxiously.

"Not right after, but I think he'll be fine after some intensive physical therapy," Dr. Forshaw replied. I let out a deep breath and tried to keep my voice steady.

"Can you have my dad call me when he wakes up from surgery? My brother can give you my number."

"Sure," he said kindly. "And if you'll just pass the message along to your mother for us . . . we spoke to her earlier, but she was pretty upset, and I'm not sure she really understood the plan."

"Oh my god, I'm so sorry about that," I apologized, embarrassed. *Note to self: don't put Mom in charge of making medical decisions if anything ever happens to me.*

"No worries," Dr. Forshaw said. "We're going to take good care of your dad. He's already taking a little nap from the anesthesia."

"Okay, thank you," I responded weakly.

I sat for a few minutes, staring at my phone's screen after it went dark. My chest felt tight and my limbs like Jello. I suddenly became aware of the adrenaline that had been coursing through my veins since I'd heard the hysteria in my mom's voice and immediately assumed the worst. When patients talked of losing their parents, like the two young men who had lost their stepfather, I was never able to imagine what it felt like. Until now. I was in my late 20s and hadn't had nearly enough time with my dad. My whole world would have collapsed. The thought of how he could have disappeared in an instant, with no warning . . . I couldn't stomach it. A strange combination of gratitude and guilt overcame me. I had been given a second chance with my dad, but others hadn't.

I also felt incredibly helpless. So what if I knew what an ORIF was? My medical knowledge and clinical experience were useless. I hadn't been at Dad's bedside, comforting him or telling him that I loved him. I couldn't be sure that he had understood the potential risks and complications when he gave consent. I would never even meet the surgeons who were putting Dad's leg back together. I was at the complete mercy of strangers and a health system that was a thousand miles away. I wished more than anything that it could have been me, instead of Eric, who was with him.

Despite his childish grumblings about the hectic hospital room environment, Eric would tell me years later that the experience ultimately shaped his perception of healthcare into a very positive one. He described how the University of Utah Hospital team attended painstakingly not only to Dad, but also to him. Both of them had arrived by ambulance in only their ski gear, and Eric was too young to drive. The medical team made sure he got a hot shower in the patient bathroom and provided him with a clean pair of PJs. Dad was NPO for surgery (nothing by mouth), but Eric got hot meals and his choice of snacks from the breakroom because the staff snuck him the code once they saw his voracious teenage appetite. They made up a bed for him on the pullout sofa in Dad's room, and checked on him while Dad was in surgery since there were no other adults around.

Eric was floored by how caring everyone was, even though he wasn't the patient. The final act that blew him away was when one of Dad's nurses drove her personal car to take them back to the ski resort, helped them collect their luggage, and returned the rental car to the airport where Mom was waiting. They had thought of everything.

Dad, too, has been eternally grateful for the incomparable care and expert skill from the healthcare professionals at the University of Utah Hospital. In those terrifying, painful, and dark days, compassion from strangers made a world of difference. It would be months before he could walk again, but the surgery was so successful that he now has more endurance than any of us on hiking trips. And more importantly, I still had a father.

TUG OF WAR

For as long as I was a PA, people always talked about work-life balance. It was possible to have it all, they said: a challenging and rewarding career, reasonable hours, job security, a family, and a social life. We simply had to create boundaries and leave work at work.

For several years, balance had seemed possible. I had my own apartment, and other than paying the bills and slowly chipping away at my student loans, my only responsibilities were to my patients. While I adored the people I worked with, I shed my professional self along with my white coat at the end of each day. Afterwards, I was just a happy, easygoing girl who enjoyed spending time with her friends, loved beautiful surroundings and glitter and soft things, and sounded like Buckbeak from Harry Potter when her real laugh came out. I laid by the pool, played trivia, had dinner with friends, hiked, read, and went to comedy shows. I relished my free time, and I was content.

Gradually and imperceptibly, work began encroaching on my personal life until one day, I realized it was just a shadow of what it used to be. Upon arriving home from an after-work meeting and eating dinner, I went straight to my laptop to login remotely and finish chart documentation. I heard Matthew say, "Baby, stop working," and I desperately wanted to, but unfinished tasks just meant additional work for me the next day. I stayed up until I had been staring at the same line for several minutes without touching a single key. After wondering why my Monday-through-Friday job simply wouldn't allow me to have a reasonable work-life balance, I finally drifted off into an exhausted but restless sleep.

Alas, I had failed to account for the great disruptor: on-call. A little past midnight, my cell phone blasted as if sending out a nationwide emergency alert. The page operator informed me that an elderly patient had chest pain. A brief conversation confirmed that he also had diaphoresis (cold sweats), shortness of breath, and dizziness. He was widowed and lived alone, so I conducted a three-way call with him and 911 so an ambulance could transport him to the ED. I'll never forget the way my own heart pounded. A few hours later, another page jolted me out of sleep, this time from a patient who hadn't had a bowel movement in three days when she usually had them daily. No red flags for obstruction or infection, just stopped up. I don't know why this registered as an urgent matter at this time of night.

The following morning, I arrived at the hospital, where I now spent the majority of my waking hours, and put out fires of varying sizes ("patient thought her appointment was today and demands to be seen now," "nurse quit yesterday and the other one is out this week," "patient is here for a vaccine appointment and we're out of stock," "insurance denied all of the patient's prescriptions.") The patient's daughter from last night's chest pain call confirmed that her father had had a heart attack; fortunately, rapid treatment at the ED had saved his life. Perhaps it was poor sleep or frustration at the lack of control over critical parts of my job duties, but I felt the crushing weight of responsibility rather than comfort. Any call could be a patient in the throes of a life-threatening emergency. Whether sleeping, driving, eating, going to the bathroom, being on call required me to be alert and to respond promptly to any of the thousands of patients in our practice. It didn't matter if I knew them or not; I was responsible for addressing them. I would obtain a brief history over the phone, log in and review the chart, and use my best clinical judgment to make a decision about their symptoms in a matter of minutes. I was on overnight call on one weeknight every week plus a 24-hour call on some weekends (more often when colleagues quit). I might get only one call during that stretch, or I might get a call every hour. If I didn't answer a page within five minutes, I could expect a second one from the hospital's answering service.

After a time, the very sound of my phone's ringtone or text message alert immediately cast a dark shroud over my spirits. It was a reminder that my job could intrude upon my personal life at any moment, and that work always took precedence. I'd scramble to find someplace quiet to answer the page; sometimes, I even pulled over on the side of the highway. It became harder to concentrate when reading, taking walks, or watching TV. I grew tired of apologizing when a page interrupted dinner with a friend, and I started declining social events because I didn't feel I could enjoy them. I'd wake up suddenly in the middle of the night and check my phone, terrified that I'd missed a page (it happened once; the colleague who was on back-up call for me was understandably very upset about being awakened). Even when I took vacations, I was frequently on call and could not fully relax or be present.

One day, I attended a seminar in which the speaker concluded that work-life balance didn't exist. We would always prioritize one or the other, she said, and trying to devote the same energy and attention to both would result in dissatisfaction. Her words were disquieting; they described my experience, which could more aptly be characterized as work-life tug of war. I was committed to the purpose of my work but also afraid I was losing myself. I was determined to honor my relationships with the people I loved, but emails, texts, and pages from work demanded my immediate response. I felt naïve and angry for believing and pursuing this illusion for so long. My work and personal life could travel next to each other in parallel, but inevitably, they would overlap. It was impossible for them to remain separate because, of course, there weren't two lives. They were just two parts of the same person's life.

After that seminar, I just kept asking myself, *How did I get here?* In retrospect, time pressure, chart tetris, the EMR, and the culture of medicine all played a role.

FIGHTING AGAINST THE CLOCK

The most pervasive feature of a clinician's day is what I call "time pressure." Although more noticeable on some days than others—and we all respond to it differently—none of us is immune once we've been practicing for some time. One urogynecologist and pelvic reconstructive surgeon, Dr. Jocelyn Fitzgerald, made a post on Twitter that gives time pressure some context:

"A non-medical friend recently asked me to describe clinic. I told her to imagine you have 20 meetings a day, half of them new clients with urgent needs. Each requires your best self. You are late for 10 of them. You must prepare a report and deliverables for each one."

After I read her words, I thought back to my own week in clinic. My meetings were back-to-back from 8:00 a.m. to 5:00 p.m. Last Saturday, I had seen almost as many patients as on a weekday, with half the time allotted (8:00 a.m. to 12:00 p.m.) and a quarter of the staff. My first patient of the morning, Ms. Ramirez, was listed on the schedule only as "New referral to OB." Innocent-sounding enough. By this stage of my career, I should have known that nothing was ever as innocuous or uncomplicated as it seemed.

Ms. Ramirez had stared at the floor throughout the entire appointment as she described how she had endured fourteen hours of labor to give birth to her first baby. He was stillborn. The pain of the contractions, however, was real and punishing.

This wasn't even the most heartbreaking part. A few weeks prior, Ms. Ramirez had seen her OB for a routine follow-up. The baby was developing as expected, but Ms. Ramirez hadn't been feeling well: congestion, facial pain, and low-grade fever. Her OB prescribed an antibiotic for acute sinusitis, assured Ms. Ramirez that it was safe to take during pregnancy, and the latter picked up the medication that same day.

Two weeks later, Ms. Ramirez felt the baby stop moving. She saw the OB urgently and nearly collapsed in the clinic when the OB realized what had happened: the label on the empty antibiotic bottle showed that the pharmacy had accidentally given Ms. Ramirez another patient's prescription. They shared the same last name and first initial. But instead of amoxicillin, the other Ms. L. Ramirez was taking methotrexate four times a week for Non-Hodgkin Lymphoma. Methotrexate is also used to terminate pregnancy, and was the reason Ms. Ramirez felt her baby stop moving at 34 weeks. Her OB advised her that labor would start spontaneously in about two weeks and that she would need to give birth even though he was already dead.

The devastating story almost brought me to tears, but somehow Ms. Ramirez stayed dry-eyed. She remained laser-focused on getting a referral from me to a new OB, even after I gently explained that it was the pharmacy, not the OB, who made the error. Ms. Ramirez maintained that forcing someone to carry a dead fetus inside for two weeks and then allowing her to scream in pain for fourteen hours of induced labor was inhumane, and she wanted nothing to do with a person who thought this was the right decision. I told her I understood.

Ms. Ramirez's appointment lasted thirty minutes instead of the allotted fifteen, and my next patient reamed me for it. I had barely made it past the doorway when she let forth a vitriol about how none of us clinicians were ever on time and how she was going to find another doctors' office to go to since we couldn't get our act together. This wasn't the first time I'd stood and faced a patient angry about my being late, but the gravity of the situation I had just been privy to made me less sympathetic. When the woman finished unleashing her wrath on me, I told her why I was late. Her features softened, and she sat down awkwardly before apologizing and telling me how embarrassed she was.

Then there was the following Monday, which always felt like getting punched in the face already, when the patient schedule had changed so much that it was entirely unrecognizable by the end of the day. *Schedule* is a misnomer, really. It is more of a rough guide: patients cancel, others take their spots, some don't show up at all, schedulers add urgent appointments, and the entire care team shuffles patients around to accommodate them if they arrive late. A countdown begins the moment we walk into a patient's room, much like sand in an hourglass. It is a continuous race against time, and its only reliable feature is its unforgiving nature. So for patients to really put themselves in their physician's or PA's shoes for a moment, I would add this to Dr. Fitzgerald's illustration of time pressure: There are no built-in breaks other than for lunch, so several times a day you decide between going to the bathroom, getting a drink of water, responding to an urgent message, or being late for your next meeting. You meet a variety of people, most of whom are nice, some of whom are extremely anxious, and some of whom are argumentative or combative. All of them expect you to be on time, and some of them tear you a new one if you aren't. Even if this is your first time meeting them, you must immediately earn their trust, and often their family's as well. You can't take a passive role in any of the meetings; you can't mute yourself, turn off your camera, or sit back and listen to what coworkers have to say. Your sole purpose is to identify problems and solve them, all while keeping an eye on the clock so that you aren't too late to the next meeting. No matter how trying your day has been or how disrespectful the other party is, you must maintain your composure and offer constructive suggestions with a smile. Sometimes you just want to drop the forced smile for a second and let yourself frown. Sometimes you get tired of pretending that everything is going great and that you don't constantly feel like you're treading water. That is the essence of time pressure.

The strain of this framework on both patients and clinicians is undeniable. Patients aren't happy about waiting, and we aren't happy about constantly running behind and apologizing for scheduling rules we don't have control over. Clinic and hospital administrators maintain that double-booking (the clinic schedules two patients for the exact same time) and/or overbooking (patients have unique appointment times, but the clinic schedules more of them overall by shortening them or creating extra slots) maximizes access to care. There will always be more patients than there are people to see them. Besides, we can't just have them stuck in limbo with no medical attention at all.

I thought of one physician I knew who had three patients scheduled for every fifteen minutes. That's right, literally five minutes per patient. Even though he saw sixty to eighty patients a day, his appointments were still booked out more than two months, and patients frequently complained about the waiting period. Aside from adding clinicians to the practice, management saw this as the only effective way to address patient demand. Were he to see fewer patients, there would be a four- to five-month wait for an appointment with him.

While PAs' schedules are typically less suffocating, double-booking is common practice, if not the rule. Even clinics that don't double-book have their own individual brands of time pressure. When I worked in urgent care, I was eligible for a bonus each quarter if I saw 3.3 patients an hour. Since we used paper charts for documentation, the sole purpose of the computers was to calculate this number as patients checked out of the clinic. One quarter, my manager gravely told me that I was ineligible for a bonus because I saw an average of only 2.9 patients an hour. I never missed a single shift, I worked weekends and holidays without complaint, and I always put forth my best effort, but my manager's only recommendation at this performance review was to increase my appointment speed so I could "hit my numbers." More appointments completed meant more charges billed and more profits. The idea that the company thought money was our main incentive for pursuing medicine was a little bleak.

I was disappointed to find that small private practices and huge public academic hospital systems, too, seemed to operate by the model of *healthcare: the business*. Monthly emails entitled "PA utilization" listed the names of each PA in our clinic alongside the number of patients he or she had seen the previous month, and the percentage of total appointments filled. I was troubled that the emails never once included the number or percentage of patients whose chronic health conditions improved from our care; the clinic did not measure or report *that* metric. Double-booking also wasn't going away; sooner appointment availability meant more reimbursement from payors.

In PA school, I remember my surprise at learning that the average amount of time a clinician listens before interrupting is seven seconds. We had all vowed to be better than that. Then we looked at our EMRs and saw two patients scheduled to see us at the same appointment time. Until a dimension existed in the universe where this was humanly possible, where was the time to actively listen to and sit with our patients? When my colleagues and I voiced our concerns or suggested scheduling and staffing changes, we were often told no by people who did not provide direct patient care, or who benefited financially from the current system. Meanwhile, we continued to struggle in time pressure quicksand, burning up our passion and energy, disappointed when we couldn't achieve the impossible. Administrators touted patient care as their priority, but for now, their slogans felt like empty words. Patient care was *our* priority.

CHART TETRIS

One evening, Matthew scooped up our dog and settled in to watch some TV while his wife reluctantly turned her attention to the other people she had professed vows to. It was a typical weekday night. I plopped myself into the desk chair in my home office to face my persistent archnemesis: Chart Tetris. This was what I called the documentation part of my job. If we don't type and sign our notes on the same day that the appointments take place, they sit there and quickly pile up on top of each other.

I scanned the shorthand I had typed during the day's appointments to jog my memory. For reference, pt = patient, RTO = return to office, h/o = history of, and ins = insurance:

8:00 a.m.
Chief Complaint #1: "My eyes hurt when sweat gets in them"
Chief Complaint #2: "I might have an STD"
   Counseled on hat vs towel. Monogamous w/wife, penile discharge and dysuria x 1 day, will RTO for results of confidential STD testing.

8:30 a.m.
Chief Complaint: Neck pain
   Pt states "I used my head to get up from the couch." No treatment.

9:00 a.m.
Chief Complaint: "I got hit by a car while I was biking"
  Advised pt to avoid biking at night, even if bike has a reflector.

9:30 a.m.
Chief Complaint: Routine 3mo Type 2 diabetes follow-up
  Pt states he was unaware of the foot ulcer I found on exam.

10:00 a.m.
Chief Complaint: Cut hand on can of red beans

10:30 a.m.
Chief Complaint: Panic attack after inspecting house and getting lost in crawl space
  No prior h/o similar symptoms.

11:00 a.m.
Chief Complaint: Med refill
  Pt checked in 20 min late for appt. No show rate 50%. Brought old RX bottle with the ink completely worn off the label. Asked what RX it was and he stated, "I don't know. But when I don't feel well, I take one and it completely knocks me out for a good 3 days. Then I wake up feeling amazing. I'm out and just need more of them."

11:30 a.m.
Chief Complaint: Tooth pain, needs root canal
  Antibiotic and referred to endodontist

1:00 p.m.
Chief Complaint: Follow-up for chronic back pain
  Appt. cut short b/c pt was arrested for falsifying RX. Stole

RX pad from doctor's office, wrote for "1 gram of mofine," and tried to fill at pharmacy. H/o opioid abuse.

1:30 p.m.
Chief Complaint: *Prior authorization needed for Botox for chronic migraine*
   Called ins. with pt present. Rep confirms all required info already in my last progress note, Botox prior auth approved. Scheduled treatment for next month.

2:00 p.m.
Chief Complaint: *Disability paperwork appeal*
   Denial reason: pt claims unable to work due to carpal tunnel and osteoarthritis in hands. Ins. found photos on her social media of her making miniature dollhouses and selling homemade wedding decorations, concluded she just didn't want to do her current job.

2:30 p.m.
Chief Complaint: *Headaches*
   Pt states "I'm at my wits' end." Noncompliant with treatment regimen.

3:00 p.m.
Chief Complaint: *Problem with birth control pills*
   Pt and boyfriend angry that RX is ineffective because she got pregnant. Side effects of abdominal pain and nausea; pt's boyfriend started taking RX after 2 months so she wouldn't have to.

3:30 p.m.
Chief Complaint: *"I can't sleep because my wife snores too loud"*

3:30 p.m. add-on
Chief Complaint: *Ingrown toenail, right big toe*

4:00 p.m.
Chief Complaint: Abdominal pain, nausea, and vomiting
   Pt's dog Piper hasn't been eating, so he ate some of Piper's food last night to convince her to eat.

4:30 p.m.
Chief Complaint: Follow-up hypertension and hyperlipidemia
   Ordered audiometry testing b/c pt had difficulty hearing his wife during visit. When she left the room, pt admitted he did not have hearing loss. He just pretends like he can't hear so he doesn't have to talk to her.
   Canceled order.

I had only completed the chart notes that involved procedures; I'd have to type out a coherent paragraph for the rest of them that included all the relevant details for whoever might read my note in the future. Indeed, it was an awesome (and exceedingly rare) day if I saw fifteen patients and finished all their notes at the end of it. Usually, a slew of administrative tasks stole my attention away every time I thought I had a few minutes to spare. "We have an administrative team that handles insurance prior authorizations so you can focus on the clinical decisions," they had told me when I interviewed for the job. Flash forward six months: the "administrative team" consisted of one brave employee who helplessly faced a deluge of incoming authorizations for our four clinicians. We might order several prescriptions or tests during a single appointment, so the inbox often had 300 new authorizations a day.

I and the other PAs quickly became the de facto second arm of the administrative team, desperately scooping water out of a sinking boat because we didn't want our one surviving support staff to quit. A typical workday consisted of me staring helplessly at a mound of insurance prior authorizations and prescription denials in my work inbox and procrastinating making phone calls with insurance companies for as long as I could. Sometimes, a live person answered after what seemed like hours of terrible hold music and automated self-service menus. There was then a 50/50 chance that I was transferred to another department or representative, to whom I begrudgingly explained why insurance should approve the medication I prescribed. I always remained polite. I knew the person on the phone was usually not the one who denied the authorization, and besides, I always treated people the way I wanted to be treated. But even the most understanding person, I would venture, becomes weary of pleading for effective and potentially life-saving treatments for patients. Optimism invariably dims when up against full-page forms and 1-800 numbers, where we defend evidence-based treatments that we've selected only after painstakingly detailing their benefits and risks in our progress notes.

Once I complete the prior auths, phone calls, messages, and problem-solving for, on average, twenty patients, I ultimately finish ten of the day's charts so I can see my family for a few hours before bed. The next day at work, the five charts from yesterday wait faithfully for me, and the next fifteen fall on top of them. If some remain incomplete by the end of the week, I will receive a warning email from my boss. Chart Tetris has no sympathy.

EMR

Like everything else that became electronic over the past decade, clinicians transitioned from writing progress notes and prescriptions by hand to typing them into EMRs. We also enter messages to staff and patients. The dilemma: there is no standard EMR in the United States; in fact, there are over 600 platforms to choose from, and every clinic might use a different one. Most aren't compatible with one another. This means patients' health information exists in bits and pieces. I can't see notes from my patient's visit to the ED last week because the hospital he went to uses a different EMR. I can't see his records from his neurologist because she also uses a different EMR and hasn't granted us access. I can't see his progress notes from his cardiologist's office because they still fax medical records instead of sending them electronically.

While EMRs should theoretically reduce documentation time because we can type faster than we can write, their redundancies and inefficiencies create a mound of busy work for us that paper charts never did. We click away on alerts and messages that pop up on the screen like a ceaseless game of Whack-a-Mole. Many EMRs don't allow us to open multiple windows at once, meaning extra steps between point A and point B, and anyone who's ever been in or worked in a medical office knows that distractions occur constantly. A single interruption can mean a prescription we forget to send or a document we forget to review. In the worst cases, it can lead to an error.

This is what happened to Taylor Lively, a 56-year-old patient who'd been coming to Sinclair Family Practice for nearly fifteen years. A hardworking and devoutly religious father of two, Mr. Lively always took his role in his health seriously and asked thoughtful questions about his potential treatments. He was someone I imagined never rushed into anything and never missed an important detail.

One day, the office manager called both my colleague, Dr. Powell, and me into her office (you'll recall that Dr. Powell is the one I ran into at the Pride parade). After she shut the door, the office manager gave us a grave look and asked if the name "Taylor Lively" rang a bell. I looked at Dr. Powell nervously; it sounded vaguely familiar, but then again, so did those of half the patients who came to the practice. The four clinicians shared care for all of them, including after-hours pages or responding to patient portal messages on one another's behalf. This was especially common for the PAs; physicians saw more patients, so we frequently completed the correspondence and tasks in their EMR inboxes. It was the actual "assistant" part of being a PA.

The office manager, Rebecca, pulled up the patient in question on her computer: 56-year-old man with hypertension, hyperlipidemia, hypogonadism, and obesity. Mr. Lively came in three to four times a year for bloodwork and follow-up, and the last time I'd seen him was about six months ago. Dr. Powell saw him for the majority of his appointments, including his most recent one a month ago.

"Oh yeah, I remember this guy," Dr. Powell said with a sigh. "He got all excited over a clerical error in the EMR, but I patched it over." He explained that in a progress note about three years ago, he had mistakenly typed *53yo WF with HTN, HLD, hypogonadism, and obesity presents for routine management.* WF was shorthand for "white female," and many clinicians copied and pasted portions of the HPI because chronic disease diagnoses were forever even if well-controlled or undetectable with treatment. With twenty patients on his daily roster, Dr. Powell was a master of using templates to reduce the amount of typing he had to do. Chart Tetris did not exist in his world; he always completed his notes on the same day that he saw the patients. I was always envious of his efficiency, and despite using a handful of templates myself, never matched his.

Dr. Powell's "insert previous HPI" template basically propagated a clerical error for much longer than it probably would have lasted otherwise. Every note thereafter began with *Taylor Lively is a [age] White female.* I mean, three years' worth. Fortunately, Dr. Powell was an excellent physician, and Mr. Lively's conditions were well-controlled. A month ago, however, Mr. Lively came in visibly upset. He demanded to know why he kept getting repeated reminders from our office about his annual mammogram. The EMR was programmed to send out these types of routine screening campaigns to all patients who met selected parameters. For breast cancer screening, the current guidelines recommended that all women aged 50-74 get mammograms. Our office had also prompted the EMR to detect relevant information from our progress notes to catch patients who might need breast cancer screening earlier; for example, women who were at higher risk because they had a strong family history. It also identified women who were older than seventy-four who were on prolonged hormone replacement therapy or already had breast cancer. The final pass-through was, of course, the clinician. We were ultimately responsible for reviewing the patient's medical history and risk factors—both could change over time—and for recommending appropriate screening. I strongly encouraged all patients to take advantage of annual wellness exams, which health insurance plans usually covered at 100 percent. Our clinic offered an array of comprehensive services including screening for breast, cervical, colon, prostate, and lung cancers; screening for diabetes, depression, and other chronic diseases; and vaccines to prevent disease.

The EMR had detected Mr. Lively's "female" status and thus sent out automatic reminders each year for mammograms. He ignored them the first two years, assuming it was meant for his wife, who was also a patient at our practice. This year, however, he read the letter more closely and noticed it was his date of birth and contact information in the heading. He checked with his wife, who confirmed that she received separate reminders on her patient portal.

"What is going on with your office?" Mr. Lively had demanded, brandishing the letter at Dr. Powell. "This is the third time you've sent me a notice for a mammogram. I know I've put on some weight, but are you saying that I have man boobs?" Dr. Powell had laughed politely, then cleared his throat when Mr. Lively didn't crack a smile and his face got progressively redder. Dr. Powell assured him that he didn't have gynecomastia, the medical term for man boobs; it was probably just a glitch in the system. Then he opened his last progress note and saw *female* in the first line. He didn't want to jump to conclusions, so he tried to casually ask what Mr. Lively's pronouns were. Perhaps that was the reason for the discrepancy in the chart. Mr. Lively did not take kindly to the question.

"He told me he was a man of God, and that God didn't make anyone a they/them," Dr. Powell recalled. "I explained that this was a standard question we ask of all patients to make sure everyone feels comfortable and respected. He didn't buy it, but I told him regardless that I fixed it in the system and it shouldn't happen again." Dr. Powell paused, apparently about to say something but deciding against it.

Rebecca wearily informed us that after a long conversation with Mr. Lively, he had chosen to stay on as a patient, on the sole condition that he did not see Dr. Powell again. He was therefore transferring his care to me. Mr. Lively understood that PAs had supervising physicians and that I communicated regularly with Dr. Sinclair. If Mr. Lively transitioned to Medicare in the future, Dr. Sinclair would likely see him for appointments since the PAs weren't contracted with them.

After everyone else went home for the day, Dr. Powell intimated to me that Mr. Lively had responded with some very homophobic things during their final interaction, and it took everything for him to resist disclosing his own identity as a gay man.

"Patients expect us to accept them exactly as they are. It's like we aren't people," he said sadly. I stood up and gave Dr. Powell a hug, which definitely seemed to surprise him, but he allowed it.

"I'm really sorry." I didn't know how else to answer.

A medical assistant once handed me a stack of unbound paper thick enough to be a book.

"The records you wanted for Mr. Weston. There's 300 pages," she told me. I stared at her, hoping she was kidding.

"These are all for one patient? And who's Mr. Weston? I don't remember ordering any medical records lately."

After a few seconds, I realized why: the date I had requested them, written across the top page, was *two years* ago. When I entered Mr. Weston's name and date of birth into the EMR, his chart displayed "inactive." He had evidently moved to a different state since his last appointment a year ago. Our office had electronically transmitted my progress notes to his new PCP; at least one party had acted in a timely fashion. I created a new task in my inbox to locate the original request for the hefty stack before me. The reason probably wasn't even relevant anymore.

I wish I could say that this kind of thing rarely happened; unfortunately, it was an all-too-familiar example of the rapid, unsystematic modernization of healthcare. In Mr. Weston's case, it was a series of EMR fails that led to a 300-page book of medical records two years past the request date. He had been hospitalized for several weeks at another facility, and although everyone there used an EMR, the medical record department inexplicably required that we fax their facility-specific form. Before I became a PA, I had assumed fax machines had died out. To my horror, I saw that not only were they still happily in operation but also as inefficient as ever and located in nearly every hallway of a billion-dollar health system. I half expected the antiquated machines to eke out that iconic '90s-era continuous form paper with the perforated edges. Hospitals and law offices might be the last two places to use fax in the current millennium. Why, I can't even fathom. Transmission is unpredictable, and a confirmation page means nothing if there is no one to review or respond to the fax on the receiving end.

Mr. Weston's chart showed that we had called the medical records department several times over the course of three months to follow up on the request I faxed. I wanted to review his diagnoses, treatments, and discharge recommendations to provide the best continuity of care possible as his PCP. We had either reached a voicemail or were told that the facility was still processing the request. A medical assistant documented after one of the calls that she *spoke to Nancy, who said the last clerk, Susannah, no longer works there. Faxed new form as requested.* She had excellent follow-through with both the facility and Mr. Weston, who sent a portal message thanking us for our continued effort to provide thorough care. Then that medical assistant quit; turnover is rampant in healthcare. We eventually hired someone, but in the meantime, all incoming faxes, referrals, and requests for records were dumped on our nurses, who were already up to their necks in direct patient care duties. Rebecca limited their allowed overtime hours to reduce staff costs, which again resulted in very disparate expectations and reality. On the one hand, complete both clinical and administrative patient tasks; on the other, patients in the clinic take precedence from 8 to 5, and max OT is fifty hours a week. Rebecca initially insisted that the nurses close encounters only once the task in question was completed, but this proved unsustainable. We had thousands of patients and hundreds of incoming documents and messages every day. Patient portals, a widespread feature of EMRs that allows secure communication with the care team, exacerbated the situation. Many patients treated them as a form of text messaging. They weren't always understanding if they did not get an immediate response from us. Most likely, we were in an exam room with another patient or on the phone with an insurance company. Even if we had a few minutes to spare before our next appointment, we couldn't guarantee an answer off the tops of our heads without reviewing a patient's notes and/or test results. We might need to reference the current literature, consult a colleague, or call up an imaging center to ask for requested test results.

    I had a love-hate relationship with the EMR, and I can only hope that electronification ultimately does more good than harm.

THE CULTURE OF MEDICINE

When I woke up one morning with a fever and vomiting, I was immediately filled with dread. An irony of choosing this profession to heal people when they are ill is that they expect us to never fall ill ourselves. On the scale of best ways to ruin everyone's day, calling in sick is second only to calling in to say you quit.

I guiltily informed our receptionist, which detonated a bomb not only in my schedule, but also my colleagues' schedules. The clinic couldn't simply cancel appointments; patients had taken off from work and other responsibilities, secured transportation, and needed timely evaluation and treatment. Postponing appointments was equally difficult because my next available one might be weeks away (for many physicians, months). The clinic therefore moved my patients to a colleague's schedule, or spread them among colleagues, all of whom already had their own appointments. They were responsible for addressing any urgent matters that came up instead of contacting me. Essentially, they were on-call for me that day. My being sick did not mean a pause in work until my return. Rather, it automatically doubled or tripled everyone else's work. Though they never said it because they were such gracious, hardworking people, my colleagues were probably aggravated. And my patients were likely angry, based on my own experience when a colleague was sick. Some were sympathetic, but many cursed or accused my colleague of being absent, unavailable, and wasting their time.

It was as if they had forgotten how bad it felt to be ill, like they were blaming us for being human.

Vacation days were an equally touchy subject because, again, a clinician's appointments for the week couldn't simply be canceled and postponed. As much as I believed that I deserved time to rest and use my work benefits just like any other employee, it always weighed on me when it came time to ask if a colleague would cover my inbox while I was out. It was an apologetic request, for the amount of work I was adding to his or her plate, even if I knew I would eventually return the favor. *Are you willing to feel like you're drowning next week?* Perhaps I would have felt like less of a monster if I had had more than two PAs I could choose between to shoulder the weight.

Guilt about asking for sick time or a vacation because of the burden it places on our colleagues seems to be specific to healthcare. If an attorney like Matthew wakes up one morning with a fever and vomiting, he can take a sick day. Staff can inform any clients who call in that he is currently out sick and will contact them upon his return. If the matter is urgent, the receptionist might consult Matthew's colleagues for advice, or him, if he isn't incapacitated. Staff and clients may grumble about the inconvenience or delay, but generally they will understand that all human beings get sick a few times a year, and that Matthew will resume his tasks when he is well.

That time, my fever and vomiting turned out to be the flu. I went to my PCP for an exam and testing, and as miserable as I felt physically, I was reassured by my diagnosis. I didn't want anyone to believe that I was feigning illness. Nevertheless, I still received one nasty note from a patient, who wrote that it was unprofessional for me to cancel his appointment without warning and pawn him off to another clinician. I learned that the office manager had told him only that I was "out of the office and unavailable" that day, not that I was sick. To appease the patient, I called and apologized for the miscommunication. He did not offer an apology of his own.

I took only three sick days in my entire ten-year career. I wore them as a badge of my dedication to my work.

PART IV

COVID-19

VOLCANO

While I had come to expect the unexpected as a PA, I certainly never imagined a pandemic just seven years into my career. I remember the early days of coronavirus disease 2019 (COVID-19) as a distant, inconspicuous rumbling—a news headline about "a cluster of cases of pneumonia of unknown etiology" that I casually overlooked. Wuhan, China first reported these occurrences to the World Health Organization on December 31, 2019. My parents planned to visit family in Beijing in January 2020.

It had been two years since Mom had seen her father, and nearly five since Dad had seen his brother. Traveling to China was no easy feat: U.S. citizens like my parents had to first drive or fly to the nearest Chinese consulate, Chicago, to apply for a $200 travel visa ($600 if an agent went on their behalf). If they were fortunate enough to receive approval and find sufficient vacation coverage at work, a one-way flight from St. Louis to Beijing cost almost a thousand dollars and took upwards of eighteen hours, including layovers. I couldn't imagine going through such an expensive, time-consuming, and unguaranteed process to see my family for only two weeks every few years. The long-awaited day in January 2020 finally arrived, and I eagerly anticipated my parents' happy reunion with my grandpa and my uncle.

Mom and Dad called a week into the trip, a phone call that will forever haunt me.

"Hey, Mom, how's the trip?" I asked brightly.

"It's good to see Grandpa . . ." She hesitated on the other end. "Emily, have you been watching the news about that virus in Wuhan? Dad and I are thinking about canceling the rest of the trip and coming home early."

"What, why?" I asked, surprised. "I thought Beijing was far away from Wuhan."

"Seven hundred miles," she affirmed, "and they've already locked down Wuhan. But even here in Beijing, all the stores are closed, and the streets are deserted. Everyone's scared that it'll be like SARS. When Dad and I walk with Grandpa around the neighborhood, it's like we're the only people in the city."

"Wow. Are y'all feeling okay?" I started pacing around my living room.

"Oh, we feel fine. We literally haven't been around anyone except Grandpa. We wear masks around him, just in case, even though he says we don't have to."

I let out a slow breath. Then Dad joined us on speakerphone. Although he told his brother and sister-in-law that he felt healthy and that there were no cases of the virus in the United States, they urged him to reconsider visiting out of an abundance of caution.

"I can tell they're scared, and I get it, so we're not going to see each other this time. At least we get to see Grandpa, so that's been worth it." Dad was trying his best to sound positive. He always put others' needs before his own, and I knew he was genuinely happy for Mom. Still, it would be excruciating for him to turn around and travel eighteen hours when he had been only a car ride away from seeing his brother for the first time in years.

Mom asked whether I thought she and Dad should curtail their trip, based on the medical facts available. I knew how much she had missed Grandpa, so she must have been really concerned if she wanted to leave him already. I pulled up Google News on my laptop and skimmed the headlines, which were largely unchanged from the week before: scientists had identified a novel coronavirus as the source of the respiratory illnesses in Wuhan, and its severity was still to be determined. Chinese citizens were worried because two other coronaviruses, SARS and MERS, had each killed almost a thousand people. However, as I explained to my parents, a new coronavirus was not necessarily a cause for alarm in and of itself. There were several coronaviruses among the more than 200 viruses that can cause a cold, otherwise known as an upper respiratory infection (URI). As a family medicine PA, I diagnosed patients with URI on a daily basis. We typically did not test for or specify which virus because most caused mild symptoms and went away without treatment. My parents were in their early 60s and in good health. Since they and Grandpa felt well, they should be okay as long as they continued to stay away from other people and to wear masks.

"You're only there for two weeks anyway," I reasoned with Mom. "You haven't seen him for two years, and it could be a long time before you see him again."

"You're right," Mom agreed, her voice sounding steadier. "I can tell he's so happy we're here. We'll just be careful, then, and keep our flight the same. Love you."

"Love you too. Tell Grandpa I said hi."

My parents returned to St. Louis in early February, jet-lagged but in good spirits. Mom had cherished her brief and long overdue reunion with Grandpa, while Dad took comfort in knowing that my uncle and aunt-in-law remained safe and healthy. There were still no cases of the coronavirus in the United States, and things almost felt back to normal. They experienced only a few small hints of what was taking place on the other side of the world. My parents' friends kindly postponed plans with them and suggested that they quarantine. Mom's employer also asked that she not come into work for another two weeks, even though she felt fine. To her surprise and pleasure, he added that she wouldn't have to use any of her PTO or sick time for this.

"This is better than getting a promotion," Mom joked to me. "I feel fine, *and* I get two weeks of real vacation."

Just days later, the United States banned the first flights from China, and the volcano that had been rumbling ceaselessly day and night erupted. Its contents spewed across China's borders, barreling across entire countries and coming ever nearer to our own. From our living room in Dallas, Matthew and I stared into the eyes of anguished and terrified Italian men and women on our TV screen. Trapped under stay-at-home orders as people died around them, they wept and begged viewers to be careful. These social media videos replayed on an endless loop, interrupted only by footage of previously unseen blue skies in heavily polluted cities in China and India, as roads and highways there became deserted. In Brazil and Columbia, drug gangs transported supplies like hand sanitizer and masks, enforced strict curfews to reduce virus transmission, and sometimes killed people who violated them. I could not process what was happening; it was like something out of a zombie apocalypse movie. There was a new name for the virus now, COVID-19, and each new case materialized like a forest fire, uncontainable and inciting more panic and terror.

Though my parents remained unharmed, my increasing knowledge about COVID-19 racked me with guilt. When I dared let myself think for even a moment about how I had convinced them to stay in China, my stomach churned, and a sour taste filled my mouth. How ignorant, shortsighted, and callous I was to think this coronavirus was just like the ones that caused the common cold! I was no epidemiologist and couldn't even call the few news articles I had read "research." My conclusions were based purely on my still paltry experience as a healthcare professional. I had reassured the people I loved most that this novel virus was probably nothing to worry about if they took reasonable precautions. My parents had trusted my medical opinion, which I had no real authority to give.

Then I learned something even worse. Mom and Dad revealed that during their stay with Grandpa, a couple and their elderly parents had lived in the apartment across the hall. The parents fell ill with COVID-19 first, followed by the couple a few days later. Within the span of two weeks, all four of them had died. As I sputtered with shock, my parents explained that they omitted these harrowing details over the phone because they didn't want to scare or worry me. Cases had not been reported outside of China, and perhaps they would remain contained so I would never have to know. They believed that sharing this information was more harmful than beneficial; after all, there was nothing I could do to protect them overseas.

When I thought about how that additional week could have cost them their lives…I tasted ash. I would have imprisoned them right in the flames of the volcano, condemned them to an inescapable fate after they had already sent me warning signals. I have regretted a lot of things I've said in the past, but never have my words so plagued me because of what I might have lost. In fact, I did not reveal these thoughts to my parents for many months, as if speaking them aloud might inflict this cursed disease upon them and take them away from me.

EARTHQUAKE

In March 2020, the pandemic became an earthquake. It rapidly gathered strength as it subsumed and devastated entire communities in its wake, as if a fault line encircled the earth. Clay Jenkins, the judge in Dallas County, issued a Shelter-at-Home order on March 23. Matthew and I had rarely watched the news before, but now, if we were awake, the TV was on. Asian, European, and Latin American faces were replaced by American ones. Numbers in the corner of the screen refreshed constantly, like perpetual ticket counter numbers, representing lives extinguished. We grew increasingly horrified as COVID-19 descended upon New York City and made it the country's worst-affected area over the course of a week. It was unreal to see once crowded and noisy streets now empty and silent as people stayed home to avoid contagion. Meanwhile, Central Park filled up with white tents because hospitals didn't have enough space to accommodate patients. When they no longer had the capacity for typical emergencies like heart attacks, trauma, and appendicitis, medical facilities turned people away. Patients died in ambulances that had nowhere to unload, and refrigerated trucks came to store dead bodies because morgues were full. Healthcare workers bravely continued caring for patients with COVID-19, even as the same sickness seized and killed them. Retired clinicians, medical students, and volunteers from other states and countries joined the deadly fight.

But the sheer number of people that COVID-19 attacked, combined with the resources and workers required to try to keep them alive, overwhelmed EDs and hospitals until the healthcare system in New York effectively collapsed.

While these images remain indelibly etched in my mind, one in particular sent aftershocks through me: aerial views showed prisoners at Rikers Island digging mass graves. Reporters claimed that New York City had paid them to bury COVID-19 victims in exchange for $6 an hour and personal protective equipment (PPE). The prisoners could still get COVID-19 since some people were contagious after death and PPE does not guarantee survival. The alternative, however, was to remain in crowded, unsanitary buildings with no capacity to quarantine and perfect conditions for infection. One inmate in the latter situation reportedly said, "We're left for dead. We're just stuck here." Perhaps those who chose the former felt the same way; the graves they dug might very well become their own. Yet this was the city's proposed solution because morgues, cemeteries, funeral homes, and even refrigerated trucks could not take any more bodies.

Of all the horrors that the pandemic had unleashed, this was by far the most terrifying. Sacrificing ourselves with no guarantee of safety seemed like one of the noblest things we could do as human beings. Those prisoners risked their lives in a time of crisis and were no different from the city's healthcare workers in this regard. Maybe they acted out of desperation, fear, or selfish desire for personal survival, but so did patients. The prisoners, though, would always be at the mercy of people who had decided that some lives were more valuable than others. COVID-19 affected everyone, bond or free, and I couldn't reconcile the invisible virus with the dark nature of humanity that it laid bare. That was the day I finally turned the TV off.

Then, just before Dallas' Shelter-at-Home order expired, an HR representative called: my employer had furloughed me for three months. I would still have a job after that, she promised, but I would not receive income or benefits in the meantime. She launched into a list of other temporary changes, which were intended to comfort me but instead struck fear into my heart. The hospital had furloughed lab researchers unless their work was directly related to COVID-19; suspended nonurgent appointments, imaging tests, and elective surgeries; and postponed clinical rotations for medical students. These were all part of its effort to prevent COVID-19 from overwhelming the hospital, the way it had in other U.S. cities like New York. Reducing personnel costs and the demand for limited PPE would redirect funding and resources to the emergency and inpatient side.

After repeating that I would not lose my job, the HR representative encouraged me to be positive and stay safe in these difficult times. Then she left me alone to contend with the uncertainty swirling around my brain. I tried to feel grateful that my job was only suspended, not gone, but I was skeptical about how the hospital could guarantee this. If there was one thing I had learned in the short time since the word *pandemic* first entered my vocabulary, it was that this was an unpredictable and constantly changing beast. I had some savings, but I didn't know if it was the equivalent of three months' salary, and I was still paying a mortgage, bills, and the minimum installment on my PA school loans. I had no major health problems, but it was terrifying to be without health insurance in the midst of a pandemic that showed no signs of stopping.

In a live online broadcast the next morning, the hospital's president echoed the sentiments of the HR representative: the implemented changes were drastic but necessary to counteract the "lost revenues in our health system and the added costs" due to COVID-19. He maintained that reducing spending by any means possible was the only way to save the jobs of all 19,000 employees and prevent the layoffs that other hospitals had resorted to. Even after freezing incomes and benefits, he woefully predicted that the hospital would "finish the fiscal year with a significant operating loss."

I didn't have any more time to dwell on the health system's potential budget deficits. All I knew was that, along with suspending my job, furlough might also suspend my livelihood. Like millions of other Americans, I filed for unemployment.

EVERY MAN FOR HIMSELF

I was one of the lucky ones. My employer stayed true to its word, and I returned to the workplace after three months. During my extended isolation at home, the only other human beings I had encountered were Matthew and a few employees at the grocery store drive-up. It was wonderful to see and talk to people again, even if it was hard to recognize them with their masks. At the same time, I was still very much afraid of getting COVID-19, bringing it home to my family, and losing coworkers or patients to the disease. I caught myself involuntarily stepping back when someone stood near me, and I barely ate half of my lunch in the breakroom the first day before yanking my mask back up. There were only two small tables where four of us sat in what now seemed like an incredibly cramped space. It was strange and unfamiliar, trying to become comfortable with physically being around other people again.

The hospital's COVID-19 measures also made me feel like I was relearning to walk. I struggled clumsily with my new N95 mask and face shield, which were required for procedures. I carefully sealed the mask in a brown paper bag at the end of each clinic session. Because of limited resources, we re-wore our N95s until they either broke or a new batch became available. I washed and sanitized my hands until the tender skin flaked and fissured at my fingertips and knuckles. I stopped wearing my white coat because it would become a breeding ground for COVID-19 particles; instead, I got in the habit of stripping down immediately upon arriving home and throwing the day's scrubs into the washer.

While I had been furloughed, hundreds of workers had materialized at each of the hospital's entrances to check everyone's temperature. Outside the employee elevators, once we passed the first screening measure with no fever, we approached computers and swiped our badges to affirm that we had not knowingly come to work with any of the COVID-19 symptoms displayed on the screens. Patients verbally answered the same set of questions at the check-in area:

> In the last week . . .
> Have you had a temperature of 99°F or higher?
> Have you had a cough, sore throat, congestion, or shortness of breath?
> Have you been around anyone who has COVID-19, or been told that you have COVID-19?

My patient, Mr. Jennings, answered "no" to all the questions when he arrived at our front desk for his follow-up. My visits with him were always enjoyable; he was a pleasant and inquisitive man, and I especially appreciated how he was always early for appointments. A wise nurse I worked with was fond of saying that "if patients are early, they're on time, and if they're on time, they're late." She was absolutely right. Time might be just a social construct, but in a medical office, a patient who arrives at 9:00 a.m. for a 9:00 a.m. appointment can unwittingly delay the entire day's structure. I was happy to learn that Mr. Jennings' headaches had been less frequent, and he seemed optimistic about the treatment plan we discussed. As I turned to leave the room, he hesitantly asked, "Emily? I have one more question."

"Sure."

"Can you order a COVID test for me?"

I nodded, sat back down, and logged in again on the EMR. "Is this for your job, or do you just want to make sure you don't have it? The system requires me to specify the reason for the test when I order it," I explained as I clicked through order sets.

"No, not for work. I've been coughing for a couple of days now, and I don't want to give it to my kids or my wife," Mr. Jennings replied.

"A couple of days?" I repeated. "I didn't notice you cough today. Have you had a fever or shortness of breath?"

"I had a fever yesterday. And I took some cough medicine before I saw you."

I frowned slightly beneath my mask as I pulled up Mr. Jennings' check-in information on the computer and confirmed his answers: *no, no, no* to having a fever, cough, or any of the other COVID-19 symptoms. Someone was in the wrong here. Our staff hadn't asked, they had selected the wrong answers on the form, or Mr. Jennings hadn't been truthful. Lying seemed out of character for him, so I gave him the benefit of the doubt and asked if he'd told us about his symptoms at check-in.

"I needed this appointment, so I told them no when they asked," he confessed, avoiding eye contact. "I meant to get tested yesterday, but things got busy at work. I figured I could just ask you when I came in today."

I felt a twinge of betrayal. It was the summer of 2020, when thirty-five people died every day in Dallas County, and 6,000 more became infected with COVID-19. Based on the devastation we'd seen over the past few months, Mr. Jennings' decisions would not just affect him. The other patients who had been sitting innocently in the waiting room, the employees I would come in contact with later that week, my husband—any one of them might be the next victim. Though I could not be sure of Mr. Jennings' intentions, I perceived an unspoken message. *I know my cough and fever mean I may have what people everywhere are dying from, but I lied because it's convenient for me.*

I want to protect my family, and I don't care if you and everyone else here gets it. This was the last thing I had expected from Mr. Jennings, and I was disappointed. I could have easily seen him for a telehealth appointment and still ordered a COVID-19 test for him, without risking anyone's life.

My job as a clinician, however, was to put my personal feelings aside and take care of the patient. I acquiesced and ordered a nasal swab for Mr. Jennings at the hospital's drive-through COVID-19 testing site. After instructing him to wear a mask and stay home until we notified him of the results, I told him sincerely that I hoped he felt better soon.

The next morning, I received his result in my inbox: positive. As required by the hospital, I reported my exposure to a patient with confirmed COVID-19 to Occupational Health. They would monitor all staff members with known contact for symptoms. I followed the call with another to Mr. Jennings. Although I didn't criticize him for lying the day before, I allowed myself to appeal to his compassionate side this time. It was still within his power to prevent harm to others by staying home and isolating until his symptoms went away. Like anyone else, he could not control what the virus did next; he could only control what *he* did next. Just as he was concerned about his wife and kids, others cared about infecting theirs. Perhaps encouraging compassion and self-reflection would save someone else from directly or indirectly getting COVID-19 from Mr. Jennings and prevent that person's disability or death. Mr. Jennings said he understood.

Not even a week later, I was again taken aback by another patient's response to the screening questions.

"Have you had any fever in the last week?" I heard Sarah, one of the front desk staff, ask as she did at least 300 times every day.

"No," a man's voice answered loudly.

"Have you had any cough or shortness of breath?"

"No to all the questions. You ask me the same thing every time," the man snapped. I looked in his direction from where I had been standing and talking to a medical assistant. The patient was a burly man with a thick, mousy brown mustache. His biceps were about to pop the seams of his short-sleeved button-up that was one size too small.

Sarah smiled and met his angry gaze with a calm one. "Yes, sir, we're in a pandemic right now, and we're doing everything we can to protect you and everyone you see here. Have you been around anyone who was diagnosed with COVID?"

The patient glared at her and stubbornly remained silent. When Sarah repeated her question in the same even tone of voice, still smiling as she said it, I thought he was going to lose it.

"NO!"

The clinic manager left her post and made her way over to check on the situation. She observed as Sarah handed the man a clipboard with a sheet of paper attached (and which he refused by folding his arms).

"I'm not answering any more of your questions," he fumed. Sarah continued to hold out the clipboard, undeterred. She was handling the unwelcome behavior remarkably.

"These are your doctor's questions," she explained. "He wants to make sure you're getting better, or find out if you're having any problems with your treatment."

Scowling, the patient finally snatched the clipboard from her. Before starting toward a chair in the waiting room, he turned to the clinic manager and gave both her and Sarah a piece of his mind.

"Healthcare is supposed to be about putting the patient first, but you guys just keep making it about you. Force us to get our temperature taken to come in and suffocate us with these masks, make us answer a bunch of questions every time.

I'm sick of it! I pay you to take care of me, not to treat me like I'm some kind of diseased criminal! Shame on you!"

The medical assistant and I retreated to our work area as the clinic manager attempted to de-escalate the situation. Just the week before, I had been blindsided by Mr. Jennings hiding his COVID-19 symptoms. Now someone was accusing us outright of serving our own interests and not caring about our patients. I understood the man's frustration. Anger, anxiety, and fear about the pandemic had been building up with no release valve, and people everywhere were coping the best they could. Some holed up at home, spraying mail and groceries with Lysol; some lashed out, defiant or in denial that this was their life now. A barrage of conflicting messages came at us each day, often changing overnight while we slept. No one enjoyed the drudgery of the hospital's rules, and it was hard to see beyond the present restrictions and mounting frustrations when the future was so uncertain. Short of banning all people from entering the building, however, screening them with temperature checks and questions about symptoms seemed like the only proactive steps the hospital could take.

At the same time, I wished I could grab the man by the shoulders and make him sit in the room with our patients who now towed oxygen tanks behind them after having COVID-19. I wanted him to talk to the families of patients younger than him who had had a stroke because of it, and ask him to still care for all the patients who had other health concerns. I was wounded that he believed we weren't putting patients first and that our toils were meaningless. Who were the people still willing to sacrifice their health—possibly their lives—every day, to attend to the pain and suffering of those who sought their help? Who honored the vows commensurate to those they gave at the altar of staying "in sickness and in health, until death do us part"? *Whose* death?

FALSE ALARM

With patients' and healthcare workers' anxiety and frustration increasing as the pandemic wore on, comic relief was in short supply in the clinic. This day looked no different when 62-year-old Mr. Hernandez came in to go over his bronchoscopy results. He'd started with a dry cough three months prior, infrequent at first but more persistent in recent weeks. When he woke up with a fever and shortness of breath, he had grown concerned that it might be COVID-19 or another virus, although he didn't know how he would have gotten it. He hadn't been around anyone for at least a month before his symptoms started. He was a retired teacher and lived alone. He had groceries delivered to his front doorstep, was religious about handwashing, and left the house only to sit in the backyard with his dog. Some distant family members had died from COVID-19, and Mr. Hernandez knew he was at higher risk because of his older age.

After two negative COVID-19 tests, he contacted our clinic and we allowed him to come in for an evaluation. I hadn't seen Mr. Hernandez since the pandemic started, and I noticed his lustrous brown hair had acquired a tinge of grey. His mind was sharp, though, and his energy as lively as ever. His history was unrevealing; he hadn't traveled anywhere in the last year, had no risk factors for TB, didn't smoke, wasn't aware of any exposure to bats, and didn't have pet birds. When I heard decreased breath sounds and spotted a hazy opacity in the right lung on a chest x-ray, I had a sinking feeling. Usually, the lungs appear black because they are filled with air. Although he did not have risk factors for lung cancer, we had discussed the possibility.

Mr. Hernandez cleared his throat nervously as he watched me login to the computer and open his chart. I had already informed him a few days after his last visit that his tests for COVID-19, the flu, RSV, and TB were all negative.

"Are you feeling okay after the bronchoscopy?" I asked, attempting to dispel some of the tension.

"Yeah, my throat was a little sore, but it's better now," Mr. Hernandez answered hoarsely. "The pulmonologist said something to me in the recovery room when I woke up from anesthesia, but I can't remember it. Maybe he was sending a sample off for testing?"

"That's pretty common. Let's take a look at the report." I kept a relaxed expression behind my mask and tried to remain positive even as my heartbeat quickened.

Suddenly, my eyes landed on the final diagnosis: FOREIGN BODY. SUNFLOWER SEED. The pulmonologist added in his note that the patient's symptoms should resolve since the seed was removed in its entirety. There was no bacterial or fungal disease. No lung cancer.

I was so overjoyed I wanted to jump up and sweep Mr. Hernandez into a bear hug. Instead, I had to remain six feet away from him per hospital rules since I was not performing a physical exam. He made me read the diagnosis aloud to him, just to be sure he had heard me correctly.

"I don't remember the last time I ate a sunflower seed," he mused. Tears moistened his eyes and then, overwhelmed with relief that neither of us had felt in weeks, we laughed.

BRAINWASHED

On a morning in the winter of 2020, I arrived at work to find one of our department's most respected and senior physicians, Dr. Morehouse, openly weeping at her desk. She had just returned from the inpatient side. All attendings were on service every few months to see admitted hospital patients, and Dr. Morehouse had been charged with caring for those who had sustained liver damage from COVID-19. After the lungs, it was the organ that took the greatest hit. While some patients went into liver failure and many died, their fates weren't the reason for Dr. Morehouse's tears.

Instead, she revealed that she was distraught over her surviving patients. Their precarious position on the verge of death had improved, in large part due to her team's meticulous around-the-clock care and strict observance of the hospital's preventative measures. Although these patients had a second chance at life, many sneered at Dr. Morehouse's requests to wear masks when she or other care team members came into the room. They said things like, "You're all brainwashed," and one patient went so far as to cough directly on Dr. Morehouse. The attending who had been on-service the two weeks prior had forewarned her of these behaviors, but Dr. Morehouse had optimistically believed she'd be able to change some of their perspectives with her experience and empathetic bedside manner. Instead, she felt helpless and discounted.

The morning of her final day on service, Dr. Morehouse woke up with a fever. As chills racked her tired, aching body, and crushing chest pain accompanied each shallow breath, she just knew. Testing confirmed that she had contracted COVID-19 from one of her patients, who had since died, and it was at that moment that her resolve crumbled. Just as her patients were confined to their hospital rooms, Dr. Morehouse had not gone anywhere for fourteen days straight except for the hospital, her car, and a hotel for hospital employees. She had not seen or touched her family, even though their hugs and kisses might have tempered the emotional and physical exhaustion of battling futilely against COVID-19 as it picked off her patients one by one. Despite taking every precaution to evade the virus, she had lost the game.

As Dr. Morehouse spent the following week in quarantine observing for worsening symptoms, her thoughts strayed toward the worst. Was she going to die now and become just another number to add to the statistics of daily deaths displayed on the news? Would she spend her final conscious moments gazing at her children, husband, and parents through a smartphone screen as she had seen some of her patients do before they passed? People with COVID-19 complications took up so much space and equipment that had to be carefully rationed. They forced ED and hospital clinicians to turn away other patients with heart attacks, strokes, and complications of cancer because there was simply nowhere to treat them. Had it been worth it, risking her life day in and day out to save people who didn't seem to care if they caused *her* death?

Dr. Morehouse felt enormously guilty for asking herself these questions. Helping patients was her life's work and sworn responsibility, but the dramatic shift she'd experienced in their attitudes and behaviors broke her spirit. At the beginning of the pandemic, patients had dutifully followed instructions to wear masks, isolate, whatever she and her team recommended if it meant possibly staying alive. Families had thanked her for risking her life to try to save their loved ones, even in cases when COVID-19 still won and left them with only grief and heartbreak. Now, they no longer seemed appreciative, but rather, disdainful or entitled. Patients (or passersby, we were still unsure) were vandalizing signs at the hospital entrance like the one that read *HEROES WORK HERE*. Dr. Morehouse was at a loss about how to cope with the pandemic's damage to the patient-clinician bond.

Several of our colleagues agreed and shared their own experiences grappling with these very personal ethical questions. Providing care for people with different beliefs and values—well, that was to be expected and part of the job description. But it was steadily becoming more difficult to maintain the same compassion, energy, and sense of duty toward patients whose convictions directly conflicted with ours. We were physically and mentally exhausted as we drew from nearly empty tanks. We comforted Dr. Morehouse as best we could before dispersing to see our own patients for the day. I busied myself with appointments and tasks, and for a time, it helped distract me.

Then Ms. Carlisle arrived. A patient in her early 40s whose feathery eyelash extensions and rich red lipstick were always on point, she sported a flowy silk caftan over skinny jeans and pointy-toed boots. She also wore a mesh face mask adorned with sequins that I immediately knew did not meet the hospital's minimum guidelines because I could see clear through it to her glossy red lips. The nurse, Serena, and I were about to perform a lengthy cyst excision on Ms. Carlisle's neck that would involve exposing ourselves to her secretions at close range.

"Ms. Carlisle, I'd like you to wear this for the procedure, please." I handed her a standard, blue, hospital-grade mask. She shook her head.

"Those blue ones are so boring! If people want to be sheep, be my guest, but that's not me." Her mask glittered like a disco ball as her lips moved, and Serena and I exchanged glances. We had started taking turns dealing with patients who resisted the hospital's mask policy, and now it was Serena's turn.

"Ma'am, we aren't asking you to throw your mask away. It's beautiful," she began in a pleasant voice.

"Thank you, I made it myself," Ms. Carlisle replied stiffly. Serena nodded.

"We just need you to protect Emily and me by wearing this for the twenty or thirty minutes you're here. Some of our staff and a lot of our patients are immunocompromised."

"But it's easier to breathe in this one," Ms. Carlisle whined.

"Yes, because it's full of holes," Serena responded without batting an eye. "COVID-19 can get through the holes, too. We promise, as soon as the procedure's over, you can put it back on."

I glanced wearily at the clock on the computer screen; this conversation was going nowhere and eating up precious minutes of our appointment. Finally, Ms. Carlisle heaved a huge sigh, groaned, and picked up one loop of the blue mask like she was holding a dead mouse by its tail. We did a time-out to confirm her name and date of birth before the procedure, and everyone in the room was just a little more irritated than when we had first walked in.

After I sketched an elliptical orbit on the skin around the cyst and injected the stinging anesthetic, I thought of all the times I had politely asked patients to please put a mask on or wear it properly so it covered the nose and mouth. The protests: *it hurts my face, I can't breathe, I hate wearing these things, masks don't work anyway, COVID is just a cold*... Rather than feeling like a healer, I felt like a soldier waging war against both an evasive and rapidly changing enemy, as well as against civilians unwilling to join forces even when they expired in vast numbers from it. Our only weapons as clinicians were our powers of persuasion and our faith that patients cared for the greater good, not just themselves. Maybe it was because I had witnessed a colleague's suffering only earlier that morning, and her raw honesty about wrestling with her conscience was still fresh on my mind.

I'm the same as you, I wanted to say to Ms. Carlisle, to all of them. I had medical training, but I didn't anticipate a pandemic and hadn't studied this disease, nor did I have any idea how to end it. Heck, maybe masking and physical distancing didn't do anything, but so far, nothing else had helped, so the best hope both patients and professionals had was to follow health authorities' recommendations. I wanted patients to understand that it wasn't about taking away their choices. Everything was a choice, except death. Patients accepted or rejected medical advice every day, whether it was agreeing to start a medicine for AFib or refusing to check blood sugar to monitor diabetes. Whereas their choices used to only affect them, they now affected anyone they came in contact with. The pandemic had become bigger than all of us. I had already seen COVID-19 destroy families, businesses, and governments. It seemed like it had also broken people's trust, both in healthcare agencies and in their fellow humans, and I worried whether that could ever be rebuilt.

AN UNEXPECTED DISCOVERY

I shut an exam room door behind me one morning, completely and utterly bewildered. I had just seen a young woman, Ms. Philips, for ear pain, which I had assumed was going to be a quick and straightforward appointment. Her history was unremarkable, but after examining her ears, I was convinced that my eyes were playing tricks on me.

I watched Dr. Sinclair emerge from a room down the hall and wave goodbye to a patient and his wife. He appeared deep in thought.

"How's your morning going, Dr. Sinclair?" I asked as he took his spot in front of a computer. I still had no idea what I was going to tell him.

"Living the dream," he responded with a soft chuckle. "This patient I just saw used to be an aircraft engineer. He has dementia now. I have to explain who I am every time I see him because he doesn't remember me, but he can still tell you how to build any part of an airplane." He shook his head with admiration. "The guy's brilliant. It's sad to see the other parts of his mind go."

"That has to be so tough," I replied. My question seemed even more insignificant now. "Dr. Sinclair . . . would you mind taking a quick look at my patient's ear? I'm very confused by what I saw on her exam."

"Sure. What's her story?" He turned his chair toward me and granted me his full attention. It was part of what made him such a great physician; he always made the other person feel like he or she was the only person whose concerns mattered.

"She's a 33-year-old woman with dull, aching, inner left ear pain for two days. No past medical history or recent trauma. No hearing loss, discharge, tinnitus, vertigo, fever, or upper respiratory symptoms. When I looked in her ear, I could see the tympanic membrane, and it was clear. But I also saw . . . letters."

"What do you mean, letters?" Dr. Sinclair repeated, furrowing his brow.

"I saw a D, an E . . . and a C, I think. It almost looked like they were just suspended in the air in the canal. I know it sounds bizarre."

Dr. Sinclair gave me an amused sideways look before standing up and following me to the exam room. He greeted the patient, got up close and personal with the otoscope, and then said to Ms. Philips with a perfectly straight face, "Ma'am, there are letters in your ear, and we need to get them out." He rooted around a drawer for a curette as Ms. Philips followed his instructions and dutifully lay down. She asked no further questions, as if this was a perfectly acceptable explanation for her ear pain.

At Dr. Sinclair's direction, I aimed a giant syringe at Ms. Philips' ear canal and forced a stream of water along the rim.

"Aha! Got it!"

Dr. Sinclair carefully maneuvered the curette and held it up to the light. He gave Ms. Philips and me a satisfied grin as he showed us a transparent sticker: MADE IN CHINA.

"Whaaaat," Ms. Philips breathed, staring at it. "How the heck did that get in my ear?"

Dr. Sinclair didn't miss a beat. "Whenever you figure it out, we want to know, too," he quipped before bidding her goodbye.

TILL DEATH DO US PART

Ms. Barrios, who saw me periodically for Crohn's disease and annual wellness exams, came in one afternoon for insomnia. Bleary-eyed and tearful, she revealed that the reason she could not sleep was that her son had unexpectedly died the week before. At only thirty years old, Rafael had been the victim of road rage after he honked at someone for cutting him off on a busy highway in Texas. The other driver sprayed bullets into his windshield, and when Rafael pulled over on the shoulder, approached and shot him in the face at point-blank range. It was broad daylight. The suspect, who was still at large, screeched away and left Rafael to bleed out like roadkill. Witnesses called 911 and tried to revive him, but it was too late.

Every time Ms. Barrios closed her eyes, she imagined Rafael's final moments, and crushing panic paralyzed her. She begged him aloud to forgive her for not being there to protect him, for letting him die vulnerable, scared, and alone. Rafael was the kindest and most peaceful person you could ever meet, she told me. He had never so much as raised his voice at anyone or held a grudge; somehow, that made the punishment of his murder even crueler. Ms. Barrios could not sleep, could not eat, could not do anything other than cry. She had cried so many tears that she thought they would dry up, but there were always more. She didn't know how she could ever bring herself to bury her only child.

We held each other in the privacy of the exam room as her

aching sobs filled the heavy air around us. Ms. Barrios and I had known each other for nearly five years, but I could never know her loss. I could only witness her grief, guilt, and anger. Many people had contracted and survived COVID-19, but death was still finding other ways to claim the lives of patients and their families.

Sometimes, the only way my colleagues and I learned that a patient had died was after we clicked on a chart and a window appeared on the screen: *[Name] is deceased. Would you still like to proceed?* We'd freeze, these few, simple words hitting us like a ton of bricks. The news might come through a phone call or portal message from a patient's family. It might arrive in the form of a death certificate for one of the physicians to sign. We'd turn to one another to express our shock because the patient seemed the picture of health the last time he or she was here, or we'd reminisce about someone we had cared for deeply over the years. We'd share tears and hugs, sometimes just a somber moment. We could not grieve for too long and neglect the living patients waiting for us in the clinic.

I learned the hard way that things were no different when we lost one of our own. One day, a patient canceled her appointment, and I gratefully settled into my office to respond to prescription refill requests with my unexpected fifteen minutes of free time. Then a medical assistant knocked on the door and extinguished my good mood with just two words: "Leila died."

Leila was one of our nurses and had seemed perfectly healthy when I talked to her just two days ago. The medical assistant sniffled as she described what had happened. When Leila did not show up for work that morning, our office manager called her house. No one answered. This was most unlike Leila, who was always punctual and rarely took a day off.

He then called Leila's emergency contact, her neighbor, who answered and was beside herself. She had heard Leila's car start every weekday morning for the past twenty-five years. That morning, she heard the car door shut as usual, but the sound of the engine didn't follow. The neighbor didn't know what it was that made her grow worried, but after ten minutes, she couldn't shake off the strange feeling and peered through the curtains in her living room. She could see Leila in the driver's seat; why was she just sitting there? The neighbor came out of the house, walked across to Leila's driveway, and waved to Jack, Leila's 6-year-old son, in the backseat. She knocked on the car window. Nothing.

Suddenly, the neighbor understood. She frantically wrenched the car door open to find Leila motionless, her skin still warm. The neighbor called 911, but she already knew. The medics pronounced Leila dead at the scene. Later, the hospital determined that she'd had a pulmonary embolism.

I could hear the medical assistant's voice, but it was as if I couldn't understand her words. Tears of anger and disbelief stung at the corners of my eyes, and my breath felt trapped in my chest, like I was going to suffocate. Energetic, talkative, and happy, Leila was everyone's best friend. She'd share a smile or a story whenever we had a break during the day. She always gave her time and attention without complaint, whether it was to her patients, her coworkers, or her child.

Jack! Who was going to take care of him? His father had been out of the picture since before Jack was even born. Leila's parents were dead, and as far as I knew, she didn't have any other family nearby.

I barely wiped away my tears before it was time for my next appointment. I was in a fog as patients detailed their various concerns to me: hair loss, sore throats, difficulty concentrating.

It all seemed so superfluous. When they looked at me expectantly for sage medical advice, I stared through them, unsure whether I had even heard them correctly or if my devastation had contorted their words. The very rise and fall of their voices were both shrill and grating to my ears. My body felt like it weighed a thousand pounds, and my face like it had forgotten how to smile. I tried to tell myself not to discount my patients' symptoms. Maybe Leila had told her PCP about a cough or chest pain or dizziness before it all happened. But the shock overwhelmed me. My thoughts were only about Leila, how she had died alone without anyone to comfort her. I hoped she had not been scared or in pain. The fact that Leila had died on her way to work somehow seemed even more unfair, and I had a constant urge to just run out of the exam room back to my office, lock myself in, and sit in the dark in silence.

My anguish intensified when I overheard the receptionist ask the office manager whether she should postpone that week's appointments for stress tests. Leila had overseen those on Mondays and Fridays.

"No, patients come first," the office manager said firmly. "I might be able to binge one of the cardiology temps from the fourth floor. Good thing it's only Tuesday. We've got time." He said this as if Leila had just taken a few days of sick leave. I knew his job was to make sure operations ran smoothly and that patients were satisfied, but he seemed so unemotional about it that my own emotions cut deeper. I was suddenly reminded of Dr. Martin's unceremonious departure after he admitted to struggling with alcohol addiction. Was that what we could expect in this profession, giving all of ourselves to relieve others of pain and suffering, only to face it alone when our own time came? A temp to fill our place so that things could be business as usual? No time, space, or permission to grieve?

Once again, death had announced itself by casting its

shadow over me. As a primary care PA, my job was to prevent disease, and by extension, early death. But the losses of Rafael and Leila weren't preventable. Death had simply robbed us of them, proving once again that all of us were completely at its mercy. I swallowed my bitter grief and managed a façade of neutrality as I went about my work, but later that week at Leila's funeral, everything I had carried inside came forth. I wept, and the tears wouldn't stop.

SAY "AHH"

I am relieved to say that all of our pediatric patients who contracted COVID-19 survived. Although I don't have any children, I felt for the parents who were at home trying to provide theirs with basic needs as well as education and entertainment. I hoped that kids would get to play together again and see one another's entire faces, and I took heart in the fact that they were so resilient. Our pediatric patients also helped lift some of the seriousness that weighed us down during the pandemic.

In February 2021, an adorable 7-year-old boy came in for his appointment dressed in a furry dinosaur costume complete with a matching face mask. He was even playing with two little stuffed animal dinosaurs while he sat in an exam room chair, and they currently appeared to be whispering secrets to each other.

"Hi, Jonah," I said with a smile. He seriously could not have been any cuter. He looked shyly up at me, then at his mom, who nodded encouragingly.

"Hi," Jonah said quietly.

"Your mom told me one dinosaur here isn't feeling good? Where is he hurting?"

Jonah hesitated, then patted his throat with a furry green paw.

"And I have a runny nose," he added.

"No fever or cough, though, and all three COVID tests this week were negative," Jonah's mom told me. "He got these dinosaurs for being such a trooper."

Poor thing. Three swabs in one week?! I'd had my fair share of ten-second countdowns while a healthcare worker twirled those stinging, eye-watering sticks up my nose. We earned ourselves a test anytime we were exposed to a coworker or patient with COVID-19, or if we had symptoms. They were awful.

Jonah seemed a little nervous about being in the clinic, so I "listened" to his dinosaurs with my stethoscope first before checking his heart and lungs.

"I'm going to look in your ears and see if there's anything in there," I explained afterward. "We'll save your nose and mouth for last, because we have to take your mask off for those."

Jonah moved his stuffed animals aside. "Okay. And I want to show you this," he said. He flipped over a sheet of paper on his lap that I hadn't noticed until now. My cheeks puffed out under my mask, and one side started to rip as I held in my laughter. On the paper was a picture of a child with brown hair and a dinosaur costume on, just like Jonah, with his eyes bulging and a tongue depressor in his open mouth. Jonah had drawn a circle around the picture and a thick red diagonal line through it.

"He drew it this morning when I told him we were coming here," Jonah's mom murmured, her eyes betraying a smile.

"I won't use the stick if you open wide enough and say 'ahh' really loud," I promised Jonah, pointing to the tongue depressor in the picture. He agreed and clutched his dinosaurs tight. Fortunately, I was able to keep my word that appointment. Jonah was so happy about avoiding the peril depicted in his drawing that he gifted it to me "in case it could help other kids." It was only a brief moment, but I laughed and had a glimpse of normalcy, what patient care used to be like and could be like again. And in that way, our kiddos gave us much-needed hope.

RICE CHASER

I generally avoided sharing personal details with patients (for example, whether I was married or had kids) to maintain a professional and neutral relationship. Preceptors had always instructed us to use our best judgment: defer or answer with the minimum relevant information, then redirect. So when patients occasionally asked me about my ethnicity, I granted a brief, polite response before moving on with the conversation.

But that was then, when such questions still surprised me because they seemed to come out of left field. No one ever asked me about my ethnicity when I was at the grocery store, walking my dog, or eating at a restaurant, after all. What was it that prompted patients to ask, and better yet, why did they assume it was an appropriate topic for a doctor's appointment? I never referenced anything Asian at work, I didn't speak any other languages, and I didn't have an accent. (I guess that last part isn't entirely true. *The New York Times'* Regional Dialect quiz concluded that my accent is from Mobile, Alabama. I've never even been to Alabama; I've just lived in Texas too long.)

I didn't believe patients meant me any harm, but I couldn't put my finger on what their intentions were, either. My colleagues had never mentioned similar experiences, and asking patients outright was the exact opposite of redirecting. I had various speculations, all of which I kept to myself. Perhaps it was a literal lack of knowledge or exposure. My particular patient demographic included people from rural towns in Texas and the surrounding states, where there were probably few Asians. Perhaps patients thought of themselves as "cultured" or inclusive by telling me about friends or family members they had who were Asian. Or perhaps they were just trying to be friendly and couldn't think of anything else to talk about.

The other issue was that I felt such a discomforting mix of emotions when people questioned my identity. I was by turns confused, embarrassed, and offended. I always checked the box *Asian or Pacific Islander* on forms, but I didn't feel Asian. I was born in St. Louis and had only lived in Missouri and Texas, so I wasn't Chinese—my parents were Chinese. Chinese American, Asian American, American Born Chinese (or ABC, as I had heard friends describe themselves) . . . all of these designations seemed needlessly complicated. I was American. I felt American and looked American. At least, I thought I did, until patients started chipping away at my sense of self by asking me where I was from. The words would clang into a conversation like cymbals next to my ears, distracting me from the legitimate clinical problems they brought to me to solve.

Matthew, who is white, joked that I should simply shut the conversation down with a far-fetched answer. You know, catch patients off their guard and signal that their question was unnecessary and insensitive.

"You should say you're from Nigeria. Or Mexico. Or say you're adopted, so you have no idea where you're from," he helpfully suggested. It was tempting, and I had to bite my tongue on many occasions. I knew those responses weren't professional, though, so I continued to answer as honestly and briefly as possible, as if it didn't bother me.

At one of his own doctor's appointments, Matthew was the one who fielded the question.

"We'll see you in six months," a staff member said as she handed him an appointment summary. I was leafing through the pages of a magazine in the waiting room and started to stand up when I overheard her next questions to him.

"Is that your wife?"

"Yes."

"Where is she from?"

The ad for incontinence underwear on the page before me suddenly became fascinating. I trained my eyes on it and kept my head down as they walked toward me.

"St. Louis," Matthew said. He knew where the conversation was headed and remained tight-lipped with his answers.

"She's so pretty," the woman replied, practically ogling at me as if I couldn't understand or see her. "What is her ethnicity?"

"Chinese."

The woman nodded knowingly and replied, "We have some Filipinos who work here."

"That's nice," Matthew said as he stood by my chair, where I sat frozen with embarrassment. At moments like this, I wanted to be invisible. He wasn't about that and put his arm around me.

"We don't know any Filipinos."

Enter the COVID-19 pandemic, and it was as if I'd undergone a pigment change in the weeks while we were holed up under Dallas' Shelter-at-Home order. Patients' "interest" in my heritage was no longer simply unwelcome; it now bordered on morbid. *The question*, or one of its infinite variations, occurred so frequently that I began to anticipate the exact moment a patient was about to ask:

"Where are you from?"
St. Louis, Missouri.
"But where are you *really* from?"

"What is your background?"
"Can I ask what your ethnicity is?"
"Where are your roots?"
"What's your heritage?"
"What is your country of origin?"
"Do you mind if I ask where your parents are from?"
"Since you're Chinese, do you speak Vietnamese, too?"

And the ones that weren't questions, merely statements:

"I'm so glad your parents came here so that you could be born here and become a PA."
"My doctors are from so many different places, it's like my team is the United Nations. And now I have a doctor from China!"

That last one finally elicited a visceral reaction from me. With a flash of anger, I retorted, "I'm not from China; I'm from Missouri. Born and raised." The patient waved his hand airily and said, "Oh, you know what I mean. I can't believe how diverse hospitals are these days."

I clenched my jaw and administered treatment for his headaches in silence. I didn't have the energy to respond, and I wasn't sure what I would say, anyway. All I knew was that the incessant questions and comments and offhanded remarks had escalated from a slight indignity to a thorn in my side. Despite my best attempts to dodge it when I saw it approaching, it'd get under my skin. I'd pull it out and try not to dwell on the soreness it left behind, but the thorn would invariably find its way back in before the sting completely disappeared. I no longer cared what patients' intentions were; I just wanted the interrogation and the scrutiny to end. I wanted people to stop implying that I was different, something to be curious or intrigued about. I barely had the bandwidth to worry about anything other than surviving COVID-19, but I had reached a dead end. It was thus that the pandemic forced me to ask myself why I had this knee-jerk reaction.

Growing up in suburban St. Louis, there had always been a handful of Asian kids in my grade. I couldn't recall a single instance in which someone asked me where I was from, or where my parents were from. I struggled to bring even two less explicit exchanges to mind.

At second-grade summer camp, I had been standing around eating my favorite summer treat, a freezer pop, when a boy I didn't know came up to my friends and me.

"Ching chang chong—what did I just say in Chinese?" he asked loudly. My friends giggled because the sounds were funny.

"Nothing," I responded, looking at the boy like he was an idiot. Didn't he know that random sounds didn't mean anything? The boy, in turn, crossed his eyes, stuck out his tongue, and ran away laughing. *Weirdo.*

A different time, a kid pulled at the outer corners of his eyes and asked, "Why do your eyes look like this?"

I shrugged, said, "That's not how they look," and skipped off. I was blissfully unaware that this is a question every Asian American gets asked at least once in his or her life. I did not dwell on the interaction for even a moment more.

Finally, there was O-Week (short for "Orientation Week") at college. Before classes start, incoming freshmen get to know each other and their residential colleges—Rice's alternative to Greek life—through a host of social activities on and off campus. I was talking, laughing, and having a good time with a cute fellow freshman in the quad until—

"My friends back home call me a 'rice chaser,' but honestly, I just think we have a real vibe," he told me, leaning in close.

"A *what*? A rice chaser?" I repeated. Maybe I'd heard wrong. Or maybe since this was Rice University, he meant he liked girls who went to school here?

"I find Asian women really attractive," he clarified. He clinked his plastic Solo cup of Keystone against the one in my hand, like we were toasting something amazing.

I stared at him wordlessly as my buzz evaporated. I had thought he was flirting with me because I was pretty or interesting, but was it really because I was... Asian? Did he look at me and see a real-life version of one of those anime cartoon characters in a miniskirt, or some exotic geisha? For the first time in my life, I felt ashamed of my appearance and trapped in my body. I was disgusted to be Asian.

"Why are you looking at me like that?" the guy asked, breaking my stunned silence. "I just told you you're attractive. You should feel flattered." He touched my shoulder lightly, and it was as if the sensation unfroze me from my daze. I made up an excuse to go find my roommates and, after they introduced me to some (normal) guys they had just met and I had another drink, I forgot all about the creepy guy and our conversation.

Maybe that was it. For the first twenty-three years of my life, almost no one had ever explicitly asked about or discussed my Asian-ness, so I'd never had to think about it. I'd dismissed the rice chaser remark as a one-off, only to feel bewildered and disconcerted when patients reintroduced my ethnicity into the conversation after I started PA school. Once the pandemic arrived, it became impossible to just forget anymore. My people were the ones buying and eating bats from wet markets in China. My face represented the source of this deadly plague that my president had nicknamed the "kung flu." Friends and family treated me like they always had, but strangers now crossed to the other side of the street when I took a walk in the neighborhood. It felt like the eyes of the nation were on anyone who remotely resembled me, and it sickened me that maybe this was the real reason patients were interested, too. This dark road of self-identity stretched far beyond shock or confusion. I started fantasizing about the impossible. At times,

I found myself wishing that I were white or black—no one would ever ask about my background again. There would be no more curiosity, ambiguity, unbelonging. The discomfort I felt in my Asian skin was indescribable. It was hell.

IT'S NOT ALL IN YOUR HEAD

It turns out there is a name for those seemingly innocent and harmless exchanges: microaggressions. Though I'd experienced them with increasing regularity since the pandemic began, I didn't hear of the term for at least two years. *Microaggression* sounded like a word the Office of Diversity, Equality, and Inclusion made up.

In a webinar over Zoom, I learned that the thorn in my side and its lingering sting wasn't all in my head or because I was overly sensitive. These statements, questions, and behaviors didn't happen to all healthcare workers. Furthermore, studies on long-term impacts consistently showed damage not only to people's physical and mental health, but also to their careers if they experienced microaggressions in the workplace. I listened in stunned silence as other healthcare professionals shared examples of microaggressions from coworkers and patients. Most were about race, but disability, gender, religion, and sexuality were also common targets.

One nurse had been alone with a patient before a procedure. She felt him watching her intently as she washed her hands and prepared to gown up. Suddenly, the patient scoffed and remarked, "Darling, you can't wash that off."

The nurse froze. She was black, and she knew at once what he was insinuating even if she'd never heard those words before. Though she was screaming inside, she said nothing, nor acknowledged the patient's comment in any way. She carefully scrubbed her hands, slowly and deliberately. As she turned off the faucet, the patient said it again, much louder this time.

"You can't wash that off."

"I was shocked and didn't want to cause any trouble, so I didn't tell the physician what happened until after the patient left," the nurse recalled. "He said he didn't tolerate racism and reported it, but his boss said we couldn't fire a patient for a 'veiled comment.' Since he didn't say 'you can't wash your blackness off' or 'you can't change the fact that you're black,' we could only send him a warning letter."

Several of the webinar's attendees shook their heads in disbelief, and a slew of sympathetic comments popped up in the chat. One of the hosts explained that a microaggression was precisely that: a veiled or subtle comment about a person's race, gender, sexuality, and so forth that causes harm. It could also be a question, attitude, or action, anything that draws attention to something different about an individual. It makes that person feel like he or she does not belong or, worse, as if his or her experience or emotions are not valid. Microaggressions reflect bias and reinforce inequality and power structures around historically marginalized groups. The people behind them are not always racist, sexist, or homophobic, nor do they necessarily have ill intentions. They may not even be aware of what they have said or done, thus, "micro" because it is not overt racism or discrimination. Yet therein lies the damage because the uncertainty (was it about my race, or something entirely unrelated?) is draining and uncomfortable. Sometimes, like the patient's comment to the nurse washing her hands, microaggressions are downright demeaning. The webinar host pointed out that referring to a nurse as "darling" was also disrespectful and sexist.

While that patient's words were almost certainly intentional and meant to get a reaction out of the nurse, an Indian-American nurse practitioner recounted an instance in which she believed a colleague's remark was unintentional, but it nevertheless had a hurtful effect.

"One of the nurses said she was proud to work on a team where several of the providers are people of color, and that patients appreciated it too. She said, 'three of our five providers are foreigners,' and gestured to me and two of the physicians. I'm from Chicago, and I've lived here my entire life. I'm not a foreigner."

Although the NP knew that her colleague meant what she had said as a compliment, the *impact* of her words mattered far more than the intentions. The microaggression was anything but micro; the nurse implied that the NP was not American, that she was an outsider. The NP still remembered her colleague's words exactly, and they still bothered her because they invalidated her identity.

An Asian physician shared an unwelcome interaction in her clinic that had occurred a few weeks after the pandemic started. Everyone was on edge and trying to get used to the new PPE and physical-distancing guidelines. One of the technicians wouldn't stop staring at her that day, and the physician finally became annoyed.

"What is it?" she asked impatiently. "Do you need help with something?"

"They say the coronavirus came from bats. Why do you people eat bats?" the technician responded, making a disgusted face.

"What do you mean, *you people?* I don't eat bats!" the physician exclaimed. Surely, this lady was joking.

"I don't know, that's just what they said on the news about coronavirus in China," the technician replied, shrugging. "You're Chinese, aren't you?"

"My coworkers almost had to restrain me. I've never been that mad at work before," the physician admitted. "I'm Chinese, but I've never known anyone there who eats bats, and of course I didn't have anything to do with COVID. I was so insulted. I only calmed down when one of my colleagues, who is African American, told me how she gets comments like that all the time. She said, 'That's the worst, when they say, *you people*.' I realized other people had it much worse than me, and I've been more outspoken when I see it happen now."

As my head reeled with these stories, the floor opened for questions. Two attendees unmuted themselves, and both admitted that they had never experienced the scenarios fellow participants had spoken of. One said he wanted to be "mindful" of his interactions in the workplace and thanked the hosts for encouraging this dialogue. I couldn't help noticing that they were both white. Had my colleagues mentioned the race of the people who made the comments in their stories? I realized it didn't matter. Any race (or gender or religion or nationality) could commit microaggressions against another—or even the same—race. Still, I hated that word, *mindful*, in that moment. It seemed like some could choose to be mindful, while subtle and overt discrimination forced it into others' daily consciousness. How much damage, I wondered, could microaggressions inflict over a lifetime? Then I remembered: *I had wished that I was white*. That is a pretty fucked-up thing to want. I had been desperate to escape my identity even when I knew it was physically impossible. It wasn't an immediate reaction; cumulative microaggressions had eroded my confidence, optimism, and trust.

If I was confused before, my emotions were even more jumbled now. Part of me was relieved: my intuition had been right that the exchanges with my patients were inherently wrong. My uncertainty and ambiguity about how to respond, about their intentions, and about whether I was just taking it too personally when they asked me the question were all typical thought processes when people experienced microaggressions. The other part of me was incredibly sad. My parents had left their families, friends, and homes behind and flown to the other side of the world where they didn't know the language or the culture so that their children could grow up in this great country. They had sworn their allegiance by becoming American citizens and changing their first names. Yet many people viewed me, an American, as a foreigner. I realized that the questions and remarks would continue, likely for the rest of my career. I had been to China three times in my life, where I was and felt, to my core, like a foreigner. I didn't belong anywhere.

IT'S IN THE AIR

None of us wanted to let Mr. Contreras go. He'd been our patient for years, and he'd become a favorite because of his charismatic personality and charming smile. He always had a compliment for everyone he encountered, whether it was the employee who kept the plants in the hospital's hallways looking like a botanical garden or a staff member whose hard work he wanted to express appreciation for. It wasn't uncommon for our medical assistants to open the door to the waiting room and find that Mr. Contreras had become friends with another patient. His joy was effortless and his energy infectious. Mr. Contreras was also a skilled carpenter and had designed a gorgeous live-edge walnut table for our breakroom as a thank you gift to the clinicians. Though twenty-some employees placed their coffees and lunches on its surface every day, its flawless glossy sheen lost none of its luster, and the hand-carved *Sinclair Family Practice* etched into one of its curves remained precisely outlined, like a secret.

Mr. Contreras' years of work as a carpenter, however, had caused significant damage to his rotator cuff, and once anti-inflammatory medications and physical therapy exercises stopped producing results, he decided to pursue surgery. Then the pandemic came, and he lost his job. He scrapped his plans for an operation once basic survival depended on his life's savings, and he was able to remain our patient only with the help of a payment plan. When Mr. Contreras' rotator cuff pain became intolerable and kept him from sleeping at night, one of the physicians in the clinic began prescribing OxyContin for him.

In the beginning, Mr. Contreras reported that 10 mg of OxyContin every 12 hours provided tremendous relief. Sometimes, just one tablet a day allowed him to go about his routine activities and even work on a few carpentry projects here or there to help pay for clinic visits. One year into the pandemic, I reviewed his chart before his follow-up appointment with me: slowly but steadily, his dose of OxyContin had increased. The initial physician had changed the prescription to 30 mg every 12 hours, and the dose was now 60 mg every 12 hours. The online Texas Prescription Monitoring Program (PMP), which we are required by law to review before prescribing controlled substances like opioids and benzodiazepines, showed that Mr. Contreras had not filled scripts from any other clinicians in Texas or the other thirty-plus states that participated in the PMP InterConnect Search. We had documented his compliance with our clinic's policies as well. He had never requested an early refill, refused any of the testing outlined by the patient-clinician controlled substances agreement, or reported losing his medication (how we loved patients' stories about prescriptions blowing out of their open car windows! It might be believable if we'd only heard it once, or if the other two prescriptions in the car weren't miraculously spared).

"Hi, Ms. Emily, you been staying healthy?" Mr. Contreras greeted me enthusiastically when I walked into the room, his eyes twinkling over his mask.

"I have. It's so nice to see you, Mr. Contreras," I responded with a smile. I felt a twinge of guilt about the information I'd already gleaned from his chart, but I listened politely as he described his refreshing sleep and improved shoulder function, thanks to OxyContin. He could be a walking commercial for it.

"Mr. Contreras, your urine tested positive for cocaine," I told him when he finished. I calmly folded my hands in my lap as I watched his face for a reaction. He looked shocked.

"That has to be a mistake!" he cried, shaking his head vigorously. "My sample must have gotten mixed up with someone else's."

"No one else has left a urine sample today," I responded quietly.

"Well, I've never done cocaine," he insisted. I wanted to believe him, I really did. Mr. Contreras was such a warm, kind-hearted soul who brought light into the clinic, especially during the dark, unremitting days of the pandemic. He remained positive even after he lost his job and his rotator cuff pain disabled him. I probably would have floundered and given up hope had I faced the same life circumstances.

I looked Mr. Contreras in the eyes. "Tell you what. I'll send your sample off for confirmatory testing. It's always possible that the result is a false positive." *Not really, though.* I knew that it was highly unlikely for another substance to show up as cocaine. I scooted towards the computer to put in the order, anyway. I wanted to display good faith.

"Ms. Emily, my girlfriend did cocaine," Mr. Contreras said suddenly, his voice louder than usual. "I didn't do any, but I was in the same room as her, so I guess I could have breathed it in from the air."

I turned and nodded solemnly, as if considering this new information. Experience had taught me that if I waited long enough, patients would often reveal the truth of their own accord. Perhaps they realized we were about to expose it and decided it would be less painful if they did instead. Mr. Contreras looked like he was going to erupt from the suspense as I stayed silent for a few moments longer. Then, he let a stream of self-incriminating words gush forth. He had tried a little bit of the cocaine. He was aware that he had violated the agreement he signed with our practice, but he'd only done it once, and he never planned to touch it again. I thanked him for being honest with me, but we both knew this was it. Our policy was immediate termination if a patient receiving prescription opioids used cocaine, and we were uncompromising on this front. Illicit drugs had no place in a treatment plan, and the combination could be deadly. A mixture of heroin and cocaine killed both Philip Seymour Hoffman and John Belushi before the age of fifty. Opioids are dangerous even when taken properly; the main cause of death is cardiorespiratory arrest because these drugs slow the breathing rate. A child who accidentally takes even one pill of OxyContin can die from an overdose.

I said goodbye to Mr. Contreras for the last time. I was as sad as anyone else to see him go.

STAPLE HIM UP

Following two horrific incidents when healthcare workers were shot to death in Texas and Oklahoma hospitals in June 2022, our department announced a live shooter training session. This turned out to be a PowerPoint presentation over Microsoft Teams during our lunch hour. A police officer and former Army Sergeant, Alexander Dunaway, nobly took on the task of preparing us for a standoff against a potential gunman. He shared wisdom and personal experience with the more than one hundred attendees: Always know where the closest exits are to your workspace and clinic rooms. If a shooter is in the building, avoid him and run first if you can. Don't hide or try to defend yourself if you can possibly get away. It was good basic advice that I wished I had received five years prior when I found myself in a potential shooter situation, huddled helplessly behind that reception desk. They hadn't taught us in PA school that we were more likely to be victims of workplace violence if we worked in healthcare than in another industry.

In today's PowerPoint, Officer Dunaway suggested strategies if we found ourselves in an exam room with the shooter on the loose outside. Lock the door, pile chairs and stools in front of it, and locate objects around you that could be used as weapons. What kinds of objects, you ask? Grab a handful of syringes and stab the shooter as many times with them as possible. Draw up sedatives and "shoot him up" with medicine, "staple him up" with a stapler, or stab him with some scissors. Both the clinician and the patient should attack the shooter because the more people that strike simultaneously, the better the chances of bringing him down.

The presentation concluded with plans for a live training session next. There was mention of simulating an attack using Nerf guns on clinicians and staff (the police department was "still ironing out the details.") I immediately pictured Styrofoam bullets flying through the halls of our hospital and being pelted while scrambling for the nearest stapler or pair of scissors. Our typical exam rooms didn't have either of these and very few instruments in general. If I were close enough to get a good staple or stab in, the gunman would certainly be close enough to blow a bullet through my brain. Maybe my best bet would be wrapping the blood pressure machine cord around his neck. I knew this was a serious and legitimate occupational hazard, but it all just felt ludicrous, like we were cartoon characters.

On a heavier note, I also realized that, in the past, my primary concern would have been that patients even considered shooting their clinicians. Now, I was learning strategies to survive in the workplace, just as little kids in elementary schools across the country were participating in active shooter drills instead of fire and tornado drills. The irony was jarring. When people get shot, they go to the hospital as patients. When patients shoot us in the hospital . . . I didn't have an answer for that. I couldn't reconcile the idea that most people choose to work in medicine to help and heal others, yet three out of four workplace violence incidents each year in the United States involve healthcare professionals. This rate is four times higher than that of other industries and "ranges from threats and verbal abuse to physical assaults and even homicide," according to the U.S. Department of Labor. And this was before the pandemic; more recent studies point to a general increase in violence toward healthcare workers since 2020.

Three months after our virtual training, Jacqueline Pokuaa, a nurse, and Katie Flowers, a social worker, were shot and killed at Methodist Dallas Hospital. This was less than fifteen minutes from where I worked, and for many, many days after, the thought crossed my mind that it could have been me. There were innumerable ways in which expectations did not match reality as a PA. I adapted to and worked through them because I believed in the continued pursuit of relief for patients' illnesses and pain. This time, the murders pushed me further away. Maybe that meant I was a coward, but I was only willing to sacrifice my life for patients, not *to* them.

RESILIENCE

Every October 6–12 is PA Week to recognize the contributions of PAs across the country and bring awareness to what we do. Most years, this week came and went at work without mention, and I didn't feel strongly either way. After all, there's a day, week, or month for everything now. PA Week was buried somewhere among National Lost Sock Memorial Day, National Pizza Week, and National Walking Month. The random week in October escaped my notice unless a colleague happened to wish me a happy PA Week.

In 2022, a new medical director came on board, and we received gift bags for PA Week for the first time: a tumbler and a badge holder with the hospital's logo, packets of lavender- and vanilla-scented stress relief lotion, and a Pocket Slider entitled *Mental Wellness* branded with the Employee Assistance Program (EAP). Curiously, I flipped this last item over and slid the card's insert into the space that read "Ways to Maintain Mental Well Being." A list of bullet points appeared in the viewing window:

- Develop a healthy, balanced lifestyle.
- Reduce stress through meditation, exercise, and regular breaks from your daily routine.
- Be realistic. If you feel overwhelmed by some activities, it is OK to say "NO!"
- Share your feelings with family and friends. Do not try to cope alone.

The pocket slider also provided information about different forms of depression and warning signs of suicide.

I appreciated the EAP's efforts to make us aware of its services; in fact, I realized that the last time I had heard anything about it was at my new employee orientation. The program provided support for personal problems at home or work like depression, anxiety, substance abuse, grief, and separation or divorce. Not all employers offered this resource, and it was available to us and our family members for free. The gift bag contents acknowledged that our work as PAs was stressful and that we could experience depression.

At the same time, the pocket slider felt like a cop-out. It echoed the same advice that I had heard ten years ago as a student: get enough sleep, nutrition, and exercise, and tell other people when you feel stressed (now with a footnote that if it became too much, we could call EAP). It referred to one of the health system's favorite buzzwords: *resilience*. Previously explained as our ability to weather and bounce back from challenges, resilience was now a catch-all term for any difficulties we encountered. The global COVID-19 pandemic was certainly not something to bounce back from. The trauma was daily and prolonged, imposing growing demands instead of time or resources for healing. The message was unchanged despite the fact that everything had changed: modes of care delivery, available resources to perform our essential job duties, patients' attitudes regarding our motivations or identities amidst a tense racial and political climate, and increasing violence toward healthcare workers.

No amount of training, of course, could have prepared us for the perseverance needed during a pandemic. But after braving the storm for two and a half years, why did it feel like we were still left to fend for ourselves? The health system seemed to reinforce a message that resilience was a personal responsibility. I had seen little concrete support or follow-up aside from flyers on cafeteria tables with the phone number for the National Suicide Prevention Lifeline. I felt like we needed so much more now that our lives were permanently divided into before COVID-19 and after COVID-19. Even as the health system promoted mental wellness, it remained silent about its practices that perpetuated or exacerbated an unbalanced workplace. Rather than taking regular breaks and saying no when overwhelmed as the pocket slider recommended, we raced to attend mandatory lunchtime and after-hours meetings, skipped lunch altogether on some days to accommodate morning patients, answered pages in the middle of the night, on days off, or for coworkers who had quit, and shared the work of fellow employees because of constant staff shortages. Managing complex diseases and acute emergencies should have been the most taxing parts of our job description. But it was everything else that tested our finite physical and emotional reserves.

Earlier in the year, I had attended a conference where a veteran physician discussed strategies to avoid burnout. He admitted that practicing medicine could be thankless work characterized by unforgiving schedules and unrealistic administrative priorities. He told us: Don't look to our bosses, but to our patients, for appreciation. We became clinicians to serve them, and when they thank us for caring and making a difference in their lives, it validates our hard work and drives us to do better. It gives us a continued or renewed sense of purpose.

Maybe he had a point, I thought to myself later. During the pandemic, when it became increasingly commonplace to learn of a patient's death or a colleague's complications from COVID-19; when I struggled through fear, frustration, and even hopelessness to put my life at risk and continue to serve my patients; when my new job duties included placating those who didn't want to wear masks and answering questions about my ethnic background, I asked myself more than once, *Why must I be the only one with unwavering compassion? Is it possible that, one day, my compassion will run out?* It wasn't that I lacked adequate compassion or empathy to begin with; I knew that much.

After some digging around, I found handwritten thank you notes I'd saved from patients over the years. In some cases, I hadn't even been aware of the impact I'd had on them until I read their kind messages. I remembered appreciating their gratitude and encouragement, and feeling happy when they were doing well. Often, their words had given me the resolve I needed to persevere with another patient's more difficult case. I reread them now. They felt especially meaningful in comparison to the PA week present from my employer, which was followed a few weeks later by a $25 gift card to Starbucks. A colleague described the gestures as "tone-deaf," and indeed, I wished they hadn't given us anything at all.

Perhaps resilience wasn't as simple as an intrinsic ability or a set of habits that helped someone be tough in the face of adversity. Guided by both our personal and collective sense of purpose, healthcare workers had continued to give our best patient care throughout the pandemic. Maybe the people who shaped our work—patients, administrators, colleagues—increased or decreased our resilience as well. They determined our time, whether the atmosphere of our workplace was respectful and supportive, and the capacity for boundaries between our professional and personal roles. Administrators selected specific metrics to quantify our effectiveness, like the monthly tally of each PA's completed appointments. They allowed implications about our impact when they opened department-wide emails with "Dear attendings, residents, medical students (and PAs) . . ." Reminding ourselves that we contributed to patients' quality of life or fewer hospitalizations, maintaining self-worth as non-physician clinicians—wasn't this already proof of our resilience? I didn't want company-branded presents or lotion. I didn't want something that oversimplified or minimized my experience. I wanted the same things from the health system that it always expected of us: kindness, compassion, and compromise. I wanted evidence that it truly understood the changing circumstances and challenges COVID-19 posed. I no longer believed that mental wellness and burnout prevention was just a personal responsibility. Employers must be equally accountable, especially in an industry which calls for its employees to put others first, be honest, and communicate effectively.

People balk at the thought of sweeping overhauls, but surely there were smaller, additive ways to bolster a system wracked by COVID. I'd worked in three outpatient clinic settings to this point, and I saw similarities in their stumbling blocks. Clinicians and staff generally grumbled for a long time before they left. Medicine is about being with patients, not speaking to them while our fingers fly over the keyboard so we can ensure our charts are closed by the end of the day. Neither is it about going into each appointment under the gun of time pressure so we can fulfill all our responsibilities as clinician, administrative assistant, researcher, and so on.

At the level of an individual clinic, it might start with eliminating double-booking and overbooking. Patient experiences and outcomes can improve when clinicians don't rush through appointments or feel irritable because they cannot see two people at the same time. Administrators would demonstrate that they not only hear, but understand, patient and clinician concerns that such practices detract from quality care, and this could repair trust within the entire system. It might involve doing away with lunchtime meetings and encouraging healthy behaviors like taking a walk or eating at a table instead of at a desk, in front of a computer, or in the car. Creating scheduled breaks, e.g. fifteen minutes during the morning and afternoon patient sessions, inserts an intentional pause in activities. These release valves could have profound effects on healthcare workers' well-being, reduce the impacts of time pressure, and possibly prevent burnout and employee turnover. Administrators devise all kinds of creative methods for us to maximize the number of patient appointments. Surely, they can apply the same time management and problem-solving for the health of their workers.

Finally, if every clinic holds a mandatory group session once a week or once a month where clinicians sit down and share their challenges, mistakes, and work stressors, participants will understand that others go through similar experiences and emotions. They will receive much-needed support from colleagues and know that they are not alone, that there isn't something wrong with them, and that it is safe to speak up. Healthcare professionals are notorious for their reluctance to seek help due to fear of repercussions and judgment. Stigma will exist as long as the system places responsibility solely on the individual. One of the physicians in my group moved to Dallas from New York. She kept up with her colleagues back home throughout the pandemic, sharing experiences, fears, and hopes with them, and bringing ideas to our clinic's operations. I believe that this professional support was at least partly responsible for her resilience. To become stronger as a team, clinicians must see that it benefits everyone to talk and hear about the traumas we witness, the pervasive stress we feel, the weight of responsibility we bear. Only we know what it is like to work in these circumstances, and just like friends and family who sustain us through them, we need an established support system at work. Never has this need been greater than since the start of the COVID-19 pandemic.

What I'm proposing is different than offering clinicians

the option to call a hotline if they feel anxious or depressed, or sending out an invitation to "join your fellow PAs for a walk at the lake this Saturday." The group sessions are not optional. They are scheduled during the workweek like any other meetings, and take place whether three or twenty clinicians are in the office that day. An EAP specialist could be present as a resource, or it could be a gathering of employees only. Ideally, these sessions would begin as part of PA and medical school curricula. By nature of their relative lack of experience, students and residents are particularly vulnerable to the medical hierarchy's rapidly shifting priorities and expectations of independent clinical judgment. They are often afraid to ask questions when problems seem insurmountable, or of speaking out when stress becomes untenable. The more closely expectations align with reality from this earliest stage in a clinician's career, the more satisfied future professionals might be with their choices. No one enjoys being surprised by what practicing medicine really entails. No one hopes to think, *if I had known it would be like this, I would have chosen differently*. We tell patients that it is common to face challenges, have questions, and need assistance. We must normalize it for those who care for them, so we can lift each other up and continue our mission.

I could no longer deny the COVID-19 pandemic's irreversible effects on the relationship between patients and clinicians, and with the health system in general. Our profession thrives on tradition—the Hippocratic oath, White Coat Ceremony, pimping, and see one, do one, teach one, among others. These traditions have to do with patient privacy, healing, learning, and service. They also existed before Google, direct messaging through patient portals, and insurance and pharmaceutical companies that hold the key to approval and payment. When technology, the breadth of medical treatment options, and the very *world* changes, healthcare has a duty to change with it. The same trait of adaptability that makes for a successful clinician makes for a successful health system.

I chose medicine, and caring for patients was very meaningful to me and gave me much happiness. I appreciated them for letting me into the most private aspects of their lives, for their honesty and courage, and for revealing much about the human condition. I can truthfully say that I gave my best self to them every day for the last ten years, and I believe I made a difference in some of their lives. But the longer I stayed, the less I recognized what it meant to practice medicine, and the less I recognized myself. And so, just as any two people in a relationship can, we grew apart.

Then I made another choice: I hung up my white coat and released all the stories that had been locked away in my head onto paper. I considered writing "on the side" while continuing to work as a PA, but deep down, I knew that this was not the way to pursue a dream. I had honored my vows to medicine. Never was this clearer than when my employer paid out my unused PTO: it was my single biggest paycheck since I had started working. My PA career had consumed my time, energy, money, and identity. Why should I give less for something that required creating?

EPILOGUE

My sabbatical from medicine was not a popular decision. My employer told me, "We don't accept your resignation," and people I loved and trusted believed I had abandoned a more worthwhile endeavor to chase a fruitless childhood dream. Some told me outright "I don't support this," while others never mentioned the book again after I described my vision. Strangers and people I barely knew were often the most encouraging and enthusiastic. Why did something that felt so right to me also feel so punishing?

But as I typed the first words that would eventually become the book you hold in your hands, I realized this same thing had already happened before. When I made that earliest pivotal choice to become a PA, someone told me that my aspiration was child's play. The irony was that, unlike many of my colleagues, I hadn't had lifelong aspirations to practice medicine that I would stop at nothing to achieve. From the time I first learned to talk, when people asked me "what do you want to be when you grow up?", I answered without hesitation that I wanted to be a writer. Every time.

I wrote indiscriminately as a child: stories, bylaws for a club I started with friends, enthralling rundowns of the day's events. *I played with Cindy after school, then had dinner with Mommy and Daddy and went to bed.* My words were honest, confident, and came easily to me. I understood the world through language. My parents allowed me to scribble about whatever crazy things my imagination yielded; they figured my enthusiasm for writing would undoubtedly make me a good doctor, lawyer, or some equally non-starving-artist profession one day.

A parent-teacher conference in second grade seemed to settle the matter. My teacher excitedly shared an over-the-top story I'd written about chocolate chip cookies, in which aromas drifted from the oven and the warm, gooey, sweet, chocolatey goodness of each bite melted in my mouth.

"Emily's a very good writer," she said, likely the only compliment she ever gave me because I was always the class troublemaker. My parents listened in amusement since I didn't even like chocolate chip cookies (my favorites are still M&M ones).

"Emily has a big imagination," they conceded. I think they knew I was extra, even as a kid. I was also determined. I would definitely be an author someday, and this chocolate chip debut was proof.

In fifth grade, my short story about our school choir made it into the local newspaper, and they even included a photo of me. In hindsight, I wished someone had asked me to supply my own because picture day photos are just brutal. But I was too busy feeling like a celebrity. The name of my elementary school was Wren Hollow, and I described how the Wren Singers performed at a local nursing home, where one of the residents clapped and bobbed her head along to each song, her face the picture of sheer delight. Her energy was infectious. Other residents and staff gradually joined in, and the Wren Singers had more fun than at any of our other performances. The line *delighted to smell such a cinnamon-y aroma* proved that not much had changed about my writing since the second grade. For now, though, I basked in in my fifteen minutes of fame.

A dose of reality finally snapped me out of my future author dream in college. I confidently turned in a paper for a poetry course after analyzing everything in the poem to a T. I even took the professor's first-day-of-class advice and asked my roommate to read my essay aloud so I could hear the unnatural, grammatically incorrect, or otherwise noncontribu-tory parts. I knew my work was good.

When the professor handed the essay back a week later, there was no letter grade, just beautiful cursive handwriting in red ink: *You noticed the trees and missed the forest. Please see me after class.* I did so sheepishly and received the professor's blunt critique in defeated silence. I was so hell-bent on analyzing every phrase and stylistic choice in the poem that I failed to capture its essence. The feedback immediately brought back memories of when my mom had obligingly read drafts of nearly all my papers in years past. (Sorry, Mom). Although English was not her first language, she had a keen sense of when I got derailed from my thesis, what she referred to as "getting carried away with" my writing. She used to help me cut out the fluff. Now, it was just me and my words. It took nineteen years for one of my teachers to finally point out that I wasn't the writer I thought I was.

The conversation with my professor motivated me to improve my craft in writing essays since they comprised most of my English assignments. But there wasn't space to do more once I chose my career. Medicine eclipsed my other dreams.

The only writing I did anymore was medical documentation, and maybe a little sporadic journaling here or there. I don't regret it, as I think that's precisely how we should pursue careers: relent-lessly. I kept my patients' thank-you notes visible to remind me of my journey as I plunged into this new territory.

I was immediately filled with gratitude at the so-called "small things" after I left the clinic. I relearned how to savor food without looking at a clock or a computer screen. I felt sunlight on my face during daylight hours again, not only fleetingly before I entered a building or parking garage. I read not only for medical edification, but for pleasure, and devoured more books in six months than I had in the last decade. Although I still have nightmares of being on call, I gradually stopped jumping every time my phone rang and became fully engaged when I was with friends and family. Eventually, I started to feel like I was in control of my own decisions again; others did not decide the value of my work with metrics. I see now that we are not meant to be limited to a single calling. We can have many passions and chase them all. We can stray from dreams and still find our way back.

It took much longer to gain perspective into how full my life had become. I flew to Phoenix, Arizona, and stood proudly by Matthew's side as the law firm he founded, Forester Haynie, was honored as one of the fastest-growing private companies in America. I hiked with friends to a wondrous place called Havasu Falls at the bottom of the Grand Canyon, where we ate fry bread and fell asleep in our tents to the sounds of rushing water. I overcame both physical and psychological challenges there, completing the final 10-mile ascent while I was sick with COVID-19 and mentally conquering my fear of heights by scaling down a vertical 200-foot cliff wall at Mooney Falls. I clung to the rockface that was slippery with mist using only chains, ropes, and faith that I would not end up dying like the man who the waterfalls were named after. I stayed with my brother for a week in Salt Lake City. Eric was five when I left St. Louis for college, and since I remained in Texas afterward, I saw him only a few times a year. We are just now getting to know each other as adults. I was able to be there when a friend brought her first child into the world; the last time we had been in the hospital together was at the beginning of her pregnancy, when she was white as a sheet and severely dehydrated from hyperemesis gravidarum. This year, I will see my 91-year-old grandpa for the first time since I became a PA. It was nearly impossible to take two or three weeks of vacation while working, much less to spend an entire paycheck on visas and plane tickets.

And of course, I had the opportunity to share this story. Of the thousands of patients I have seen throughout my career, many have left indelible impressions. They taught me about far more than health and illness. They showed me the range of the human heart and its capacity for love, pain, hope, humility, and understanding. Whether in life or death, they deserve to be seen and heard as people, not just as numbers or names or dollar signs. The same is true for the healthcare workers who continue to make it their life's work to heal others, regardless of the sacrifice. I have witnessed tenacity and bravery beyond anything that we could learn in PA school. I will remember the kindness of classmates, colleagues, mentors, and friends that allowed for the laughter and the joy of healing. Whether from a patient, a clinician, or a stranger on the street, kindness costs nothing and can be everything to its recipient.

APPENDIX
PHOTOS

Customs-Meeting Others

- **Chinese** - Slight bow
  - Handshake acceptable
  - Use proper titles
- **Japanese** - Long low bow
  - Never use first name
- **Korean** - Bow and shake with both hands
  - Men through doors first
- **Vietnamese** – hands together at chest and bow
  - Younger person bows first

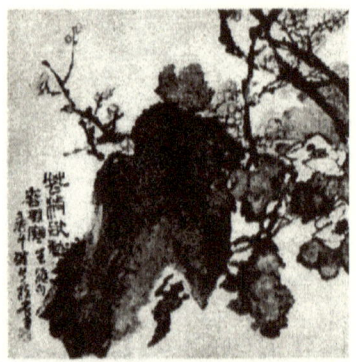

Slide from Cultural Competency lecture on Traditions: Asian Americans.

PART I | DIDACTIC YEAR: CULTURAL (IN)COMPETENCY

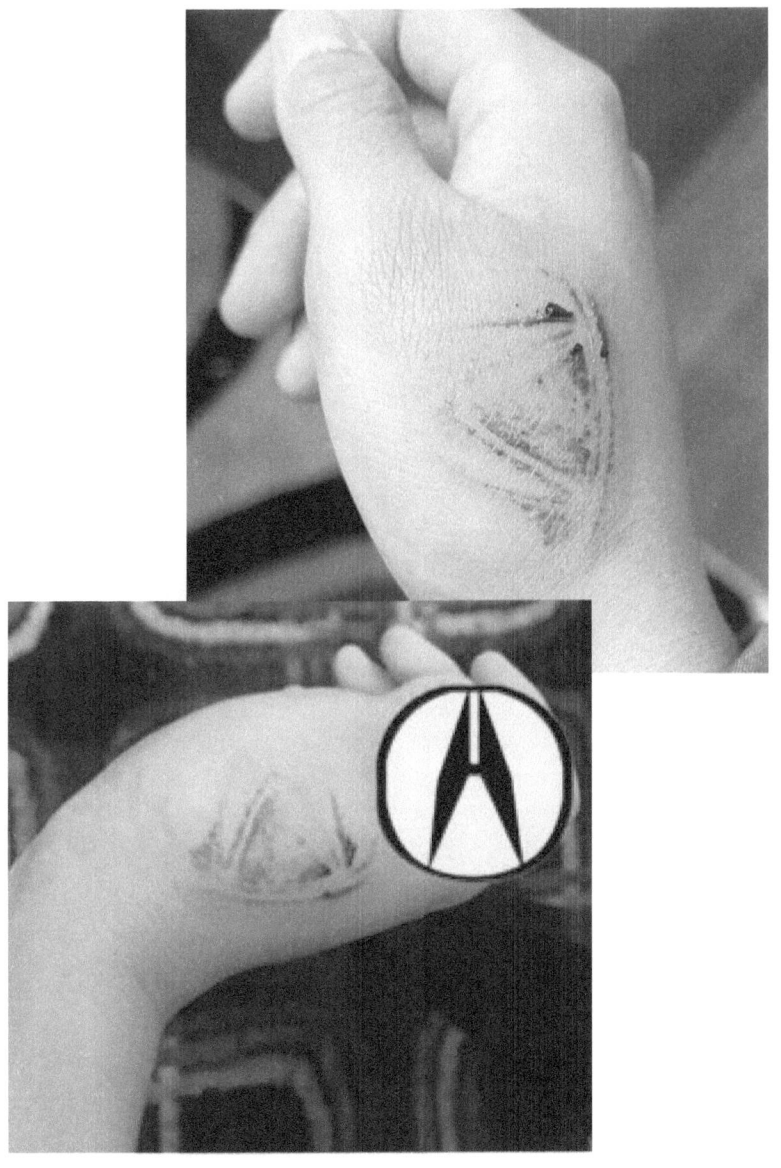

Photo of hand tattoo from Acura airbag following an MVA.

PART III | THE SPARK

1. Shares information from meetings and seminars with staff ■ ☐
2. Accessible to staff and a visible role model ■ ☐
3. Gives clear instructions and communicates necessary information ■ ☐
4. Follows up on assignments to ensure that work is completed ■ ☐
5. Interacts with home office and other ▬▬ locations in order to provide continuity of care ■ ☐

COMMENTS:
Is very accessible to the staff and communicates well. Always completes assignments and follows up. Work on presenting herself more as a leader than as a peer.

SCHEDULES   YES   NO
1. Responsible to work scheduled shifts as assigned ■ ☐
2. If unable to work, finds replacement ■ ☐
3. If unable to find replacement, contacts immediate supervisor ■ ☐
4. Reports to work promptly – five minutes before starting shift ■ ☐

COMMENTS:
Is very flexible with the schedule. Shows up to all her shifts.

TEAMWORK   YES   NO
1. Works cooperatively within own department and within other areas ■ ☐
2. Willingly accepts additional responsibility – tries to make others' job easier ■ ☐
3. Helps room and discharge patients as needed according to policy ■ ☐
4. Coordinates with others to plan and implement changes ■ ☐
5. Maintains at least 3.3 patients/hour *Goal is 3.3 or higher* ☐ ■

COMMENTS:
Willing travels to help out other clinics. Helps nurses discharge and helps lab run tests. Has been below 3.0 at times, this is usually when the volume of patients is lower. Average pt per hour this year is 2.9. Rooming her own patients when the nurses are behind would help the clinic run smoother as well as help increase her pts per hour. *Discharge your own pts when busy to help give the nurses more time to room. You should be at 3.3 pts/hr.*

Performance review in which seeing 3.3 patients/hour qualifies each PA for a bonus

PART III | FIGHTING AGAINST THE CLOCK

Other Stresses

Ways to Maintain Mental Well Being

Ways to Prevent Postpartum Depression

Seasonal Affective Disorder (SAD)

Medication

Depression & Gender

Manic Depression

Psychotherapy

The first step toward dealing with depression is determining how you're really feeling.

The following statements were adapted from the test devised by Dr. William Zung of Duke University to assess your general depression level.

- I feel downhearted, blue, and sad.
- Morning is when I feel the best.
- I have crying spells, or feel like it.
- I have trouble sleeping at night.
- I eat as much as I used to.
- I don't enjoy being looked at, talked to, or being with attractive women or men.
- I notice that I'm losing weight.
- I have trouble with constipation.
- My heart beats faster than usual.
- I get tired for no reason.
- My mind is as clear as it used to be.
- I find it easy to do the things I used to do.
- I am restless and can't keep still.
- I feel hopeful about the future.
- I am more irritable than usual.
- I find it easy to make decisions.
- I feel that I am useful and needed.
- My life is pretty full.
- I feel that others would be better off if I was dead.
- I still enjoy the things I used to.

The statements are only a guideline to assess your symptoms and do not constitute a clinical diagnosis.

- Develop a healthy, balanced lifestyle.
- Reduce stress through meditation, exercise, and regular breaks from your daily routine.
- Be realistic. If you feel overwhelmed by some activities, it is OK to say "NO!"
- Share your feelings with family and friends. Do not try to cope alone.

PocketSlider™

How To Use This Guide:
1. Place guide inside palm with fingers and thumb gently gripping outer edges of guide.
2. Gently pull tab with other hand until inside card slides smoothly.
3. Pull tab until dot lines up on desired topic.
4. View reference tips in cut out window.

Mental wellness pocket slider from Employee Assistance Program.

PART IV | RESILIENCE

> Dear Ms. Haynie,
> I wanted to write you a personal note to thank you for your hard work. I appreciate your good bed side manner and determination to find something that works for me. Its nice to have a DR. that truly cares about you. I'm grateful that you are caring for my migraines.

Thank you note from a patient.

PART IV | RESILIENCE

Dear Dr. Zhu,

I wanted to express my gratitude to you for your medical expertise in 2016. My lab results at that time indicated that I had Hepatitis C from transfusions that were performed in the 70's and 80's. Of course, I was in the panic mode when I saw you in the office that day. You reassured me that I would be fine and that all I needed was a Hepatitis A injection and Harvoni treatments. I made an appointment with Dr. ▇▇▇▇ and he too, reassured me. Upon your advice, my husband was tested (which came back negative) and he received a Hepatitis A injection. Dr. ▇▇ also reassured me when I saw him. I completed my treatments in eight weeks. My lab results since then have indicated "Not Detected". I can finally exhale. After 45 years of teaching, I now have a new outlook as I face retirement.

You have become very "special" to me as we bond. You helped me to realize that each day starts a new chapter in this journey we call, "Life". Edwin Markham once said, "There is a destiny that makes us friends. None goes his own way alone. All that we send into the lives of others comes back into our own."

I once read that there are twelve things to remember in life: The Value of Time; The Success of Perseverance; The Pleasure of Working; The Dignity of Simplicity; The Worth of Character; The Power of Kindness; The Influence of Example; The Obligation of Duty; The Wisdom of Originality; The Virtue of Patience; The Improvement of Talent and The Joy of Love. What a beautiful blueprint for life.

In the years ahead, I hope that you continue being the best doctor that you can be. I feel so fortunate to have crossed your path in life. Thank you for being there.

Thank you note from a patient.

PART IV | RESILIENCE

Students Share Fun Times With Favorite Older Adults

Young people have a great ability to capture life's funny moments. When the humor has to do with beloved seniors, their tales can be downright delightful—mainly because young persons are so tickled when seniors slip up or act silly. You can sense their thrill upon learning that normally care-worn older adults can be kid-like too!

This month, students in the upper grades at Parkway Southwest Middle School in West County shared stories of humorous times with older adults. The following three students won first place in this month's writing contest:

The Warblers and The Nightingale

By Emily Zhu

On a chilly afternoon in December, the scents of Christmas greeted Wren Hollow's "Wren Singers" outside a nursing home. Delighted to smell such a cinnamony aroma, the members tuned their voices to the right pitch. Our director, Mrs. Gruber, giggled as we warbled away. She then organized us into groups, and we filed into the build-

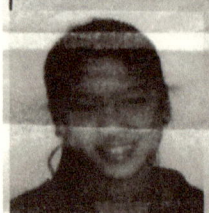

Emily Zhu

Excerpt from "The Warblers and The Nightingale".

EPILOGUE

ACKNOWLEDGMENTS

Matthew, the moment you made it real was when you placed my manuscript in my hands, with me as Nelly for the cover illustration. Without you, these stories would have stayed locked away in my head. Your enthusiasm, support, and off-the-cuff titles and punchlines are unrivaled. You truly see and understand my vision.

Holly, you generously devoted your time and skill to the many iterations of this book. You taught me the value of the writing process and the patience it deserves, and you transformed my dream into a reality. It is one thing to have talent and wisdom; it is another to make it your life's work to share it with others. I will forever be indebted to you.

Meagan, you gave my manuscript life with beautiful cover and formatting work. Thank you for your patience as I made changes at the eleventh hour.

Ann and **Andrea**, thank you for embracing my idea of this book and speaking it into existence. Our friendship is one of the things I am most grateful in from my career. You walked beside me every day (literally!) and are phenomenal at everything you set your mind to.

Christina, thank you for your infinite kindness and encouragement since they first assigned us to be physical examination partners. You taught me that our paths are not straight but full of winding twists and turns. That is precisely the incredible thing about life.

Hannah, words are inadequate for your tireless dedication to your patients and their families, your sacrifices, and your strength. Thank you for the wonderful book recommendations as I embarked on this project. You will always be one of my biggest inspirations, and I look forward to the many amazing things you still have yet to do.

Jordan, thank you for making the time to read those early drafts. Even though they were a hot mess, you provided honest but gentle feedback, and this version is all the better for it.

Eric, you believed that this was worthwhile even if our aspirations in life could not be more different. When you were younger, you once told me you could never work in healthcare because what I did was so boring. Hopefully, I've changed your mind about the latter.

Mom and **Dad**, you have made so many sacrifices for me and have never given up on me. You modeled and cultivated integrity and compassion, and I strive to make them my most defining traits.

Kyial, you came into my life at the perfect time. Thank you for being one of my greatest champions; I'm no J.K. Rowling, but I still managed to become a writer :) You constantly awe me with your selflessness and courage.

Emilia, **Leanna**, and **Willow**, you were the first brave souls to read drafts of my stories. Thank you for lifting me up as a fellow writer.

Thank you to everyone at **Forester Haynie** for supporting and encouraging me.

Thank you to all my supervising physicians, and especially **Dr. Ross** and **Dr. Henry**, for your tireless mentorship and for having so much heart. You have changed the lives of so many people, including mine.

To **every PA, physician, nurse, medical assistant, technician, administrative assistant,** and **patient** I have ever worked with, thank you for allowing me to share your stories. Special thanks to my fellow PAs who supplied ideas online, made me laugh, and lent your support to this endeavor. Without you, this book would not exist.

Emily Haynie, PA-C